Fourth Edition

Registered Health Information Technician (RHIT) Exam Preparation

Darcy Carter,
MHA, RHIA

and

Patricia Shaw,
MEd, RHIA, FAHIMA

Editors

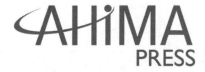
PRESS

ISBN: 978-1-58426-385-2

AHIMA Product Number: AB105012

AHIMA Staff:
Jessica Block, MA, Assistant Editor
Jill S. Clark, MBA, RHIA, Technical Review
Kathryn A. DeVault, RHIA, CCS, CCS-P, Technical Review
Angela Dinh Rose, MHA, RHIA, CHPS, Technical Review
Julie A. Dooling, RHIT, Technical Review
Katherine Greenock, MS, Editorial and Production Coordinator
Jason O. Malley, Director, Content Creation and Development
Diana M. Warner, MS, RHIA, CHPS, Technical Review
Pamela Woolf, Managing Editor

**For more information, including updates, about AHIMA Press publications, visit
http://www.ahima.org/publications/updates.aspx**

American Health Information Management Association
233 North Michigan Avenue, 21st Floor
Chicago, Illinois 60601-5809
ahima.org

Contents

On the Website

Practice Questions and Answers

Practice Exam 1 and Answers

Practice Exam 2 and Answers

Practice Exam 3 and Answers (*Bonus Exam*)

Health Information Management Glossary—Electronic Flashcards (4,500+ terms)

Hospital Statistical Formulas Used for the RHIT Exam

About the Editors

Darcy Carter, MHA, RHIA, earned her master's degree in healthcare administration and is currently pursuing a doctorate degree in health sciences. She is on the faculty in the health information management and technology programs at Weber State University, where she teaches courses in coding, reimbursement, and database management. Ms. Carter also continues to work as a coder/abstractor at McKay-Dee Hospital Center.

Patricia Shaw, MEd, RHIA, FAHIMA, earned her master's degree in education in 1997 and is currently working on a doctorate degree in education. Ms. Shaw has been on the faculty of Weber State University since 1991 where she teaches in the health information management and health services administration programs. She has primary teaching responsibility for the quality and performance improvement, coding, reimbursement, and data management curriculum in those programs. Ms. Shaw maintains contact with practice settings as a consultant specializing in the areas of reimbursement and coding issues. Prior to accepting a position at Weber State University, Ms. Shaw managed hospital health information services departments and was a nosologist for 3M Health Information Systems.

About the RHIT Exam

Professionals who hold the RHIT credential are health information technicians who ensure the quality of medical records by verifying their completeness, accuracy, and proper entry into computer systems. They may also use computer applications to assemble and analyze patient data for the purpose of improving patient care or controlling costs. RHITs often specialize in coding diagnoses and procedures in patient records for reimbursement and research.

Although most RHITs work in hospitals, you will also find them in a variety of other healthcare settings including office-based physician practices, nursing homes, home health agencies, mental health facilities, and public health agencies. In fact, employment opportunities exist for RHITs in any organization that uses patient data or health information such as pharmaceutical companies, law and insurance firms, and health product vendors.

The National Commission for Certifying Agencies (NCCA) has granted accreditation to AHIMA's Registered Health Information Technician (RHIT) certification program. This accomplishment establishes AHIMA as the industry leader in accredited health information and informatics management (HIIM) certification programs, and advances AHIMA's organizational mission of positioning AHIMA members and certificants as recognized leaders in advancing professional practice and standards in HIIM.

The Commission on Certification for Health Informatics and Information Management (CCHIIM) manages and sets the strategic direction for the certifications. Pearson Vue is the exclusive provider of AHIMA certification exams. To see sample questions and images of the new exam format, visit ahima.org/certification.

For more detailed RHIT exam information, including eligibility requirements, visit ahima.org/certification.

RHIT Exam Competency Statements

A certification exam is based on an explicit set of competencies. These competencies have been determined through a practitioners' job analysis study. The competencies are subdivided into domains and tasks, as listed here. The exam tests only content pertaining to these competencies. Each domain is allocated a predefined number of questions at specific cognitive levels to make up the exam.

Domain I: Data Analysis and Management (20% of exam)

1. Abstract information found in health records (for example, coding, research, physician deficiencies, etc.).
2. Analyze data (for example, productivity reports, quality measures, health record documentation, case-mix index).
3. Maintain filing and retrieval systems for health records.
4. Identify anomalies in data.
5. Resolve risks and/or anomalies of data findings.
6. Maintain the master patient index (for example, enterprise systems, merge/unmerge medical record numbers, etc.).
7. Eliminate duplicate documentation.
8. Organize data into a useable format.
9. Review trends in data.
10. Gather/compile data from multiple sources.

11. Generate reports or spreadsheets (for example, customize, create, etc.).
12. Present data findings (for example, study results, delinquencies, conclusion/summaries, gap analysis, graphical).
13. Implement workload distribution.
14. Design workload distribution.
15. Participate in the data management plan (for example, determine data elements, assemble components, set timeframe).
16. Input and/or submit data to registries.
17. Summarize findings from data research/analysis.
18. Follow data archive and backup policies.
19. Develop data management plan.
20. Calculate healthcare statistics (for example, occupancy rates, length of stay, delinquency rates, etc.).
21. Determine validation process for data mapping.
22. Maintain data dictionaries.

Domain II: Coding (18% of exam)

1. Apply all official current coding guidelines.
2. Assign diagnostic and procedure codes based on health record documentation.
3. Ensure physician documentation supports coding.
4. Validate code assignment.
5. Abstract data from health record.
6. Sequence codes.
7. Query physician when additional clinical documentation is needed.
8. Review and resolve coding edits (for example, correct coding initiative, outpatient code editor, National Coverage Determination, Local Coverage Determination, etc.).
9. Review the accuracy of abstracted data.
10. Assign POA (present on admission) indicators.
11. Provide educational updates to coders.
12. Validate grouper assignment (for example, MS-DRG, APC, etc.).
13. Identify HAC (hospital-acquired condition).
14. Develop and manage a query process.
15. Create standards for coding productivity and quality.
16. Develop educational guidelines for provider documentation.
17. Perform concurrent audits.

Domain III: Compliance (16% of exam)

1. Ensure patient record documentation meets state and federal regulations.
2. Ensure compliance with privacy and security guidelines (HIPAA, state, hospital, etc.).
3. Control access to health information.
4. Monitor documentation for completeness.
5. Develop a coding compliance plan (for example, current coding guidelines).
6. Manage release of information.
7. Perform continual updates to policies and procedures.

8. Implement internal and external audit guidelines.
9. Evaluate medical necessity (CDMP—clinical documentation management program).
10. Collaborate with staff to prepare the organization for accreditation, licensing, and certification surveys.
11. Evaluate medical necessity (outpatient services).
12. Evaluate medical necessity (data management).
13. Responding to fraud and abuse.
14. Evaluate medical necessity (ISSI (utilization review)).
15. Develop forms (for example, chart review, documentation, EMR, etc.).
16. Evaluate medical necessity (case management).
17. Analyze access audit trails.
18. Ensure valid healthcare provider credentials.

Domain IV: Information Technology (12% of exam)

1. Train users on software.
2. Maintain database.
3. Set up secure access.
4. Evaluate the functionality of applications.
5. Create user accounts.
6. Troubleshoot HIM software or support systems.
7. Create database.
8. Perform end user audits.
9. Participate in vendor selection.
10. Perform end user needs analysis.
11. Design data archive and backup policies.
12. Perform system maintenance of software and systems.
13. Create data dictionaries.

Domain V: Quality (12% of exam)

1. Audit health records for content, completeness, accuracy, and timeliness.
2. Apply standards, guidelines, and/or regulations to health records.
3. Implement corrective actions as determined by audit findings (internal and external).
4. Design efficient workflow processes.
5. Comply with national patient safety goals.
6. Analyze standards, guidelines, and/or regulations to build criteria for audits.
7. Apply process improvement techniques.
8. Provide consultation to internal and external users of health information on HIM subject matter.
9. Develop reports on audit findings.
10. Perform data collection for quality reporting (core measures, PQRI, medical necessity, etc.).
11. Use trended data to participate in performance improvement plans/initiatives.
12. Develop a tool for collecting statistically valid data.
13. Conduct clinical pertinence reviews.
14. Monitor physician credentials to practice in the facility.

Domain VI: Legal (11% of exam)

1. Ensure confidentiality of the health records (paper and electronic).
2. Adhere to disclosure standards and regulations (HIPAA privacy, HITECH Act, breach notifications, etc.) at both state and federal levels.
3. Demonstrate and promote legal and ethical standards of practice.
4. Maintain integrity of legal health record according to organizational bylaws, rules and regulations.
5. Follow state mandated and/or organizational record retention and destruction policies.
6. Serve as the custodian of the health records (paper or electronic).
7. Respond to Release of Information (ROI) requests from internal and external requestors.
8. Work with risk management department to provide requested documentation.
9. Identify potential health record related risk management issues through auditing.
10. Respond to and process patient amendment requests to the health record.
11. Facilitate basic education regarding the use of consents, healthcare power of attorney, advanced directives, DNRs, etc.
12. Represent the facility in court related matters as it applies to the health record (subpoenas, depositions, court orders, warrants).

Domain VII: Revenue Cycle (11% of exam)

1. Communicate with providers to discuss documentation deficiencies (for example, queries).
2. Participate in clinical documentation improvement programs to ensure proper documentation of health records.
3. Collaborate with other departments on monitoring accounts receivable (for example, unbilled, uncoded).
4. Provide ongoing education to healthcare providers (for example, regulatory changes, new guidelines, payment standards, best practices, etc.).
5. Identify fraud and abuse.
6. Assist with appeal letters in response to claim denials.
7. Monitor claim denials/over-payments to identify potential revenue impact.
8. Prioritize the work according to accounts receivable, patient type, etc.
9. Distribute the work according to accounts receivable, patient type, etc.
10. Maintain the Chargemaster.
11. Ensure physicians are credentialed with different payers for reimbursement.

RHIT Exam Specifications

The RHIT exam lasts 3½ hours and is made up of 150 four-option, multiple choice questions. ICD-9-CM, CPT, and HCPCS coding concepts are tested; however, no code books are needed to take the RHIT exam. All necessary information needed to answer coding questions is included. During the exam, formulas for commonly used healthcare rates and percentages will be provided only for items for which they are needed. These formulas are also listed on page 250 in the back of this book. A calculator will also be available during the exam. For the most up-to-date RHIT exam information, visit ahima.org/certification.

How to Use This Book and Website

The RHIT practice questions and exams in this book test knowledge of content pertaining to the RHIT competencies published by AHIMA.

The multiple choice practice questions and practice exams in this book and accompanying website are presented in a similar format to those that might be found on the RHIT exam. This book contains 520 multiple choice practice questions and two complete practice exams organized by the RHIT domains. (Each practice exam contains 150 questions.) Because each question is identified by one of the seven RHIT domains, you will be able to determine whether you need knowledge or skill building in particular areas of the exam domains. Pursuing answer references will help you build your knowledge and skills in specific domains.

To effectively use this book, work through all of the practice questions first. This will help you identify areas in which you may need further preparation. For the questions that you answer incorrectly, read the associated references to help refresh your knowledge. After going through the practice questions, take one of the practice exams. Again, for the questions that you answer incorrectly, refresh your knowledge by reading the associated references. Continue in the same manner with the second exam and third practice exam. (Practice Exam 3 is a bonus exam on website only.)

The accompanying website contains the same 520 practice questions and two practice exams printed in the book and a bonus practice exam. Each of the self-scoring exams can be run in practice mode—which allows you to work at your own pace—or exam mode—which simulates the 3½-hour timed exam experience. The practice questions and simulated exams on the website can be presented in random order, or you may choose to go through the questions in sequential order by domains. You may also choose to practice or test your skills on specific domains. For example, if you would like to enhance your skills in domain II, you may choose only domain II questions for a given practice session. You may retake the practice exams as many times as you like.

The accompanying website also includes electronic flashcards for more than 4,500 health information management-related terms as well as a listing of commonly used formulas for the RHIT exam that are available to test takers during the exam.

PRACTICE QUESTIONS

Start: 10:07 am   finish 11:08 am (watching t.v.)

Domain I Data Analysis and Management

1. A critical early step in designing an EHR is to develop a(n) _____ in which the characteristics of each data element are defined.

    a. Accreditation manual

    b. Core content

    c. Continuity of care record

    d. Data dictionary

2. Once hospital discharge abstract systems were developed and their ability to provide comparative data to hospitals was established, it became necessary to develop:

    a. Data sets

    b. Data elements

    c. Electronic data interchange

    d. Bills of mortality

3. In healthcare, data sets serve two purposes. The first is to identify data elements to be collected about each patient. The second is to:

    a. Provide uniform data definitions

    b. Guide efforts toward computerization

    c. Determine statistical formulas

    d. Provide a research database

4. A health information technician is responsible for designing a data collection form to collect data on patients in an acute-care hospital. The first resource that she should use is:

    a. UHDDS

    b. UACDS

    c. MDS

    d. ORYX

5. Which of the following is *not* a characteristic of the common healthcare data sets such as UHDDS and UACDS?

    a. They define minimum data elements to be collected.

    b. They provide a complete and exhaustive list of data elements that must be collected.

    c. They provide a framework for data collection to which an individual facility can add data items.

    d. The federal government recommends, but does not mandate, implementation of most of the data sets.

6. In a paper-based system, the completion of the chart is monitored in a special area of the HIM department called the _____ file.

    a. Incomplete record

    b. Permanent

    c. Temporary

    d. Remote storage

7. Consider the following sequence of numbers. What filing system is being used if these numbers represent the health record numbers of three records filed together within the filing system?

   36-45-99

   37-45-99

   38-45-99

   a. Straight numerical
   b. Terminal-digit
   c. Middle digit
   d. Unit

8. The MPI is necessary to physically locate health records within the paper-based storage system for all types of filing systems, *except*:

   a. Alphabetical
   b. Middle-digit
   c. Termination-digit
   d. Straight numerical

9. The RHIT supervisor for the filing and retrieval section of Community Clinic is developing a staffing schedule for the year. The clinic is open 260 days per year and has an average of 600 clinic visits per day. The standard for filing records is 60 records per hour. The standard for retrieval of records is 40 records per hour. Given these standards, how many filing hours will be required daily to retrieve and file records for each clinic day?

   a. 6 hours per day
   b. 10 hours per day
   c. 15 hours per day
   d. 25 hours per day

10. In which of the following systems are all encounters or patient visits filed or linked together?

    a. Serial numbering system
    b. Unit numbering system
    c. Straight numerical filing system
    d. Middle-digit filing system

11. Which of the following is a disadvantage of alphabetical filing?

    a. Easy to train new personnel to file
    b. Uneven expansion of file shelves or cabinets
    c. Ease of creation
    d. Relies on an index or authority key

12. Which of the following is a request from a clinical area to check out a health record?

    a. Outguide folder
    b. Requisition
    c. MPI
    d. Patient registry

13. Which of the following statements describes alphabetical filing?

    a. File the record alphabetically by first name, followed by the last name alphabetically and then alphabetically by middle initial.

    b. File the record alphabetically by the last name, followed by alphabetical order of the first name, and then alphabetical order of the middle initial.

    c. File the record alphabetically by the last name, followed by the middle initial and then the first name.

    d. File the record alphabetically by last name only.

14. In analyzing the reason for changes in hospital's Medicare case-mix index over time, the analyst should start with which of the following levels of detail?

    a. Account level

    b. MS-DRG level

    c. MDC level

    d. MS-DRG triples, pairs, and singles

15. Which of the following tools is usually used to track health records that have been removed from their permanent storage locations?

    a. Deficiency slips

    b. Master patient indexes

    c. Outguides

    d. Requisition slips

16. What is the term that is used to mean ensuring that data are not altered during transmission across a network or during storage?

    a. Media control

    b. Integrity

    c. Mitigation

    d. Audit controls

17. Which of the following filing methods is considered the most efficient?

    a. Alphabetical filing

    b. Alphanumeric filing

    c. Straight numeric filing

    d. Terminal-digit filing

18. The primary purpose of a minimum data set in healthcare is to:

    a. Recommend common data elements to be collected in health records

    b. Mandate all data that must be contained in a health record

    c. Define reportable data for federally funded programs

    d. Standardize medical vocabulary

19. In long-term care, the resident's care plan is based on data collected in the:

    a. UHDDS

    b. OASIS

    c. MDS

    d. HEDIS

20. Incorporating a workflow function in an electronic information system would help support:

    a. Tasks that need to be performed in a specific sequence

    b. Moving patients from point to point

    c. Registration of patients

    d. Making computer output available to laser disk

21. An audit of a hospital's electronic health system shows that diagnostic codes are not being reported at the correct level of detail. This indicates a problem with:

    a. Data granularity

    b. Data consistency

    c. Data comprehensiveness

    d. Data relevancy

22. Each of the three dimensions (personal, provider, and community) of information defined by the National Health Information Network (NHIN) contains specific recommendations for:

    a. Government regulations

    b. Core data elements

    c. Privacy controls

    d. Technology requirements

23. A core data set developed by ASTM to communicate a patient's past and current health information as the patient transitions from one care setting to another is:

    a. Continuity of Care Record

    b. Minimum Data Set

    c. Ambulatory Care Data Set

    d. Uniform Hospital Discharge Data Set

24. The home health prospective payment system uses the _____ data set for patient assessments.

    a. HEDIS

    b. OASIS

    c. MDS

    d. UHDDS

25. The data set designed to organize data for public release about the outcomes of care is:

    a. UHDDS

    b. DEEDS

    c. MDS

    d. HEDIS

26. Which of the following allows a user to insert, update, delete, and query data from a database?

    a. C++

    b. C

    c. Java

    d. SQL

27. Which of the following indexes and databases includes patient-identifiable information?

    a. MEDLINE

    b. Clinical trials database

    c. Master patient/population index

    d. UMLS

28. A notation for a diabetic patient in a physician progress note reads: "Occasionally gets hungry. No insulin reactions. Says she is following her diabetic diet." In which part of a problem-oriented health record progress note would this be written?

    a. Subjective

    b. Objective

    c. Assessment

    d. Plan

29. A notation for a hypertensive patient in a physician ambulatory care progress note reads: "Blood pressure adequately controlled." In which part of a problem-oriented health record progress note would this be written?

    a. Subjective

    b. Objective

    c. Assessment

    d. Plan

30. Which of the following provides a standardized vocabulary for facilitating the development of computer-based patient records?

    a. Current Procedural Terminology

    b. Healthcare Common Procedure Coding System

    c. *International Classification of Diseases, Ninth Revision, Clinical Modification*

    d. Systematized Nomenclature of Medicine Clinical Terminology

31. Which of the following provides a system for classifying morbidity and mortality information for statistical purposes?

    a. Current Procedural Terminology

    b. *Diagnostic and Statistical Manual of Mental Disorders,* Fourth Revision

    c. Healthcare Common Procedure Coding System

    d. *International Classification of Diseases, Ninth Revision, Clinical Modification*

32. What is the difference between data and information?

    a. Data represent basic facts, whereas information represents meaning.

    b. Data are expressed in numbers, whereas information is expressed in words.

    c. Information must be kept confidential, whereas data are meant to be shared.

    d. Information is about people, whereas data are about things.

33. Information standards that provide clear descriptors of data elements to be included in computer-based patient record systems are called _____ standards:

    a. Vocabulary

    b. Structure and content

    c. Transaction

    d. Security

34. Given the following file numbers, which are arranged correctly in terminal-digit filing order?

    a. 43-42-00
       52-43-00
       64-55-01
       70-41-00

    b. 43-42-00
       64-55-00
       70-41-00
       52-43-01

    c. 70-41-00
       43-42-00
       64-55-00
       52-43-01

    d. 52-43-01
       43-42-00
       64-55-00
       70-41-00

35. Dr. Jones entered a progress note in a patient's health record 24 hours after he visited the patient. Which quality element is missing from the progress note?

    a. Data completeness

    b. Data relevancy

    c. Data currency

    d. Data precision

36. Mrs. Smith's admitting data indicates that her birth date is March 21, 1948. On the discharge summary, Mrs. Smith's birth date is recorded as July 21, 1948. Which quality element is missing from Mrs. Smith's health record?

    a. Data completeness

    b. Data consistency

    c. Data accessibility

    d. Data comprehensiveness

37. Which of the following is used to plot the points for two variables that may be related to each other in some way?

    a. Force-field analysis

    b. Pareto chart

    c. Root cause analysis

    d. Scatter diagram

38. The HIM data analytics professional is reviewing a chart (shown here) on nosocomial infections presented by the hospital's infection control committee. The committee is reporting that the decrease in infection rate has accelerated over the past 10 years. What comments should the data analytics professional make?

Nosocomial Infection Rate by Year									
0.20									
0.15									
0.10									
.09									
0.07									
0.06									
0.05									
0.04									
0.03									
0.02									
0.01									
	1950	1960	1970	1980	1982	1990	1995	2000	2005

Infection rate

    a. Concur with the conclusion of the committee.

    b. State that the greatest decrease in infection rate in a year took place in 2005.

    c. State that the greatest decrease in infection rate occurred in 1960 and 1970.

    d. Request a new data chart be presented that accurately reflects the trend of infection rate.

39. Which of the following is a primary weakness of the paper-based health record?

    a. Difficult to provide availability to a number of providers at the same time

    b. Poor communication tool

    c. Difficulty in documenting healthcare processes

    d. Lack of available resources

40. Which of the following elements is *not* a component of most patient records?

    a. Patient identification

    b. Clinical history

    c. Invoice for services

    d. Test results

41. Which of the following is *not* a characteristic of high-quality healthcare data?

    a. Data relevancy

    b. Data currency

    c. Data consistency

    d. Data accountability

42. City Hospital's HIM department made a decision to discontinue outsourcing its release of information (ROI) function and perform the function in house. Because of HIPAA implementation, the department wanted better control over tracking release of information. Given the graph shown here, how would you evaluate the ROI revenue growth?

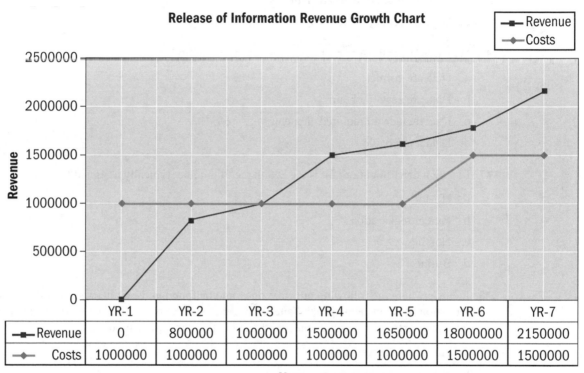

Release of Information Revenue Growth Chart

	YR-1	YR-2	YR-3	YR-4	YR-5	YR-6	YR-7
Revenue	0	800000	1000000	1500000	1650000	18000000	2150000
Costs	1000000	1000000	1000000	1000000	1000000	1500000	1500000

Year

    a. The ROI function continues to cost more than revenues generated.

    b. Annualized revenue for YR-7 is more than the costs

    c. The ROI function costs are inversely related to revenue generated.

    d. The ROI costs for YR-7 are greater than the revenue.

43. Which of the following represents an example of data granularity?

    a. A progress note recorded at or near the time of the observation

    b. An acceptable range of values defined for a clinical characteristic

    c. A numerical measurement carried out to the appropriate decimal place

    d. A health record that includes all of the required components

44. Which of the following is a primary purpose of the health record?

    a. Document patient care delivery

    b. Regulation of healthcare facilities

    c. Aid in education of nurses and physicians

    d. Assist in process redesign

45. Which of the following best describes data comprehensiveness?

    a. Data are correct

    b. Data are easy to obtain

    c. Data include all required elements

    d. Data are reliable

46. Which of the following best describes data accessibility?

    a. Data are correct

    b. Data are easy to obtain

    c. Data include all required elements

    d. Data are reliable

47. In which department or unit is the health record number typically assigned?

    a. HIM

    b. Patient registration

    c. Nursing

    d. Billing

48. Identify where the following information would be found in the acute-care record: "Following induction of an adequate general anesthesia, and with the patient supine on the padded table, the left upper extremity was prepped and draped in the standard fashion."

    a. Anesthesia report

    b. Physician progress notes

    c. Operative report

    d. Recovery room record

49. Identify where the following information would be found in the acute-care record: "CBC: WBC 12.0, RBC 4.65, HGB 14.8, HCT 43.3, MCV 93."

    a. Medical laboratory report

    b. Pathology report

    c. Physical examination

    d. Physician orders

50. The attending physician is responsible for which of the following types of acute-care documentation?

    a. Consultation report

    b. Discharge summary

    c. Laboratory report

    d. Pathology report

51. A nurse is responsible for which of the following types of acute-care documentation?

    a. Operative report

    b. Medication record

    c. Radiology report

    d. Therapy assessment

52. Which of the following is an example of clinical data?

    a. Admitting diagnosis

    b. Date and time of admission

    c. Insurance information

    d. Health record number

53. The following is documented in an acute-care record: "HEENT: Reveals the tympanic membranes, nares, and pharynx to be clear. No obvious head trauma. CHEST: Good bilateral chest sounds." In which of the following would this documentation appear?

    a. History

    b. Pathology report

    c. Physical examination

    d. Operation report

54. A hospital is concerned about the difficulty in retrieving health records for patient care and legal purposes. Some of its data are stored electronically while the remainder are stored on paper. The hospital knows it will be several years before it will be able to implement an entire EHR system and go paperless. Given this information, which of the following would be the best solution for the hospital to ensure that all of the data for a patient data are retrieved when needed?

    a. Continue with the current system

    b. Implement a document scanning system for storage of the paper record

    c. Implement a microfilm system for storage and retrieval of the paper records

    d. Implement a document scanning system for the paper records and interface data created in the current EHR with the document scanning system

55. The following is documented in an acute-care record: "Atrial fibrillation with rapid ventricular response, left axis deviation, left bundle branch block." In which of the following would this documentation appear?

    a. Admission order

    b. Clinical laboratory report

    c. ECG report

    d. Radiology report

56. The following is documented in an acute-care record: "Spoke to the attending re: my assessment. Provided adoption and counseling information. Spoke to CPS re: referral. Case manager to meet with patient and family." In which of the following would this documentation appear?

   a. Admission note

   b. Nursing note

   c. Physician progress note

   d. Social service note

57. Which of the following materials is *not* documented in an emergency care record?

   a. Patient's instructions at discharge

   b. Time and means of the patient's arrival

   c. Patient's complete medical history

   d. Emergency care administered before arrival at the facility

58. In a problem-oriented health record, problems are organized:

   a. In alphabetical order

   b. In numeric order

   c. In alphabetical order by body system

   d. By date of onset

59. Which of the following best describes an integrated health record format?

   a. Each section of the record is maintained by the patient care department that provided the care.

   b. Integrated health records are intended to be used in ambulatory settings.

   c. Documentation is integrated and arranged in alphabetical order by documentation type.

   d. Documentation from various sources are integrated and arranged in strict chronological order.

60. Which of the following represents documentation of the patient's current and past health status?

   a. Physical exam

   b. Medical history

   c. Physician orders

   d. Patient consent

61. Which of the following contains the physician's findings based on an examination of the patient?

   a. Physical exam

   b. Discharge summary

   c. Medical history

   d. Patient instructions

62. What is the function of a consultation report?

   a. Provides a chronological summary of the patient's medical history and illness

   b. Documents opinions about the patient's condition from the perspective of a physician not previously involved in the patient's care

   c. Concisely summarizes the patient's treatment and stay in the hospital

   d. Documents the physician's instructions to other parties involved in providing care to a patient

63. Which of the following is a secondary purpose of the health record?

   a. Support for provider reimbursement

   b. Support for patient self-management activities

   c. Support for research

   d. Support for patient care delivery

64. Use of the health record by a clinician to facilitate quality patient care is considered:

   a. A primary purpose of the health record

   b. Patient care support

   c. A secondary purpose of the health record

   d. Policy making and support

65. In designing an electronic health record, one of the best resources to use in helping to define the content of the record as well as to standardize data definitions are standards promulgated by the:

   a. Centers for Medicare and Medicaid Services

   b. American Society for Testing and Measurement

   c. Joint Commission

   d. National Center for Health Statistics

66. Messaging standards for electronic data interchange in healthcare have been developed by:

   a. HL7

   b. HEDIS

   c. The Joint Commission

   d. CMS

67. The HIM department is planning to scan non-electronic medical record documentation. The project includes the scanning of health record documentation such as history and physicals, physician orders, operative reports, and nursing notes. Which of the following methods would be best to help HIM professionals monitor the completeness of health records during a patient's hospitalization?

   a. Ad hoc scanning

   b. Concurrent scanning

   c. Retrospective scanning

   d. Post-discharge scanning

68. Using a hospital discharge database, a physician does a study of diabetes mellitus comparing age of onset with response to a specific drug regimen. The physician has gathered _____ from the database.

    a. Data elements

    b. Information

    c. Informatics standards

    d. Data sets

69. Two clerks are abstracting data for the same case for a registry. When their work is checked, discrepancies are found. Which data quality component is lacking?

    a. Completeness

    b. Validity

    c. Reliability

    d. Timeliness

70. Which of the following terms refers to the incidence of death?

    a. Classification

    b. Morbidity

    c. Mortality

    d. Vital statistics

71. Review of disease indexes, pathology reports, and radiation therapy reports is part of which function in the cancer registry?

    a. Case definition

    b. Case-finding

    c. Follow-up

    d. Reporting

72. Cancer registries receive approval as part of the facility cancer program from which of the following agencies?

    a. American Cancer Society

    b. National Cancer Registrar's Association

    c. National Cancer Institute

    d. American College of Surgeons

73. Which of the following is a database from the National Health Care Survey that uses the patient health record as a data source?

    a. National Health Provider Inventory

    b. National Ambulatory Medical Care Survey

    c. National Employer Health Insurance Survey

    d. National Infectious Disease Inventory

74. Which of the following contains a list maintained in diagnosis code number order for patients discharged from a facility during a particular time period?

    a. Physician index

    b. Master patient index

    c. Disease index

    d. Operation index

75. Which of the following contains a list maintained in procedure code number order for patients discharged from a facility during a particular time period?

    a. Physician index

    b. Master patient index

    c. Disease index

    d. Operation index

76. Case finding is a method used to:

    a. Identify patients who have been seen or treated in a facility for a particular disease or condition for inclusion in a registry

    b. Define which cases are to be included in a registry

    c. Identify trends and changes in the incidence of disease

    d. Identify facility-based trends

77. In a cancer registry, the accession number:

    a. Identifies all the cases of cancer treated in a given year

    b. Is the number assigned to each case as it is entered into a cancer registry

    c. Identifies the pathologic diagnosis of an individual cancer

    d. Is the number assigned for the diagnosis of a cancer patient entered into the cancer registry treatments and at different stages of cancer

78. Vital statistics include data on:

    a. Research projects in which new treatments and tests are investigated to determine whether they are safe and effective

    b. Births, deaths, fetal deaths, marriages, and divorces

    c. Medicare claims

    d. ICD diagnoses codes

79. The most prevalent trend in the collection of secondary databases is:

    a. Increased use of encryption technology

    b. Increased use of encoders

    c. Increased use of automated data entry

    d. Widespread implementation of electronic medical records

80. A record is considered a primary data source when it:

    a. Contains information about the patient that has been documented by the professionals who provided care to the patient

    b. Contains data abstracted from a patient record

    c. Includes data stored in a computer system

    d. Contains data that are entered into a disease-oriented database

81. The following data were derived from a comparative discharge database for hip and femur procedures:

Comparative Data on Hip and Femur Procedures for Current Year				
	Hospital A	Hospital B	Hospital C	Hospital D
Hip procedures	2,300	1,467	2,567	1,100
Femur procedures	988	1,245	1,067	678

These data can best be described as:

    a. Aggregate data

    b. Identifiable data

    c. Patient specific data

    d. Primary data

82. Suppose that there are six males and 14 females in a class of 20 students with the data reported as 3/1. What term could be used to describe the comparison?

    a. Ratio

    b. Percentage

    c. Proportion

    d. Rate

83. In a frequency distribution, the lowest value is 5 and the highest value is 20. What is the range?

    a. 5 to 20

    b. 15

    c. 7.5

    d. 20 to 5

84. What is the mean for the following frequency distribution: 10, 15, 20, 25, 25?

    a. 47.5

    b. 20

    c. 19

    d. 95

85. Suppose that 5 patients stayed in the hospital for a total of 27 days. Which term would be used to describe the result of the calculation 27 divided by 5?

    a. Average length of stay

    b. Total length of stay

    c. Patient length of stay

    d. Average patient census

86. Which of the following statements best describes the difference between a hospital inpatient and a hospital outpatient?

    a. Outpatients are treated in the emergency department; inpatients receive services in the regular clinical departments of the hospital.

    b. Inpatients always stay in the hospital overnight; outpatients never do.

    c. Inpatients receive room, board, and continuous nursing services in areas of the hospital where patients generally stay overnight; outpatients receive ambulatory diagnostic and therapeutic services.

    d. Outpatients primarily receive diagnostic services; inpatients receive mostly therapeutic services.

87. Given the numbers 47, 20, 11, 33, 30, 30, 35, and 50, what is the mode?

    a. 30

    b. 32

    c. 32.5

    d. 35

88. What is (are) the format problem(s) with the following table?

Community Hospital Discharges by Sex		
Sex	Number	Percentage
Male	3,000	37.5%
Female	5,000	62.5%
Unknown	—	—
Total	8,000	100%

    a. Title is missing.

    b. Variable names are missing.

    c. There are blank cells.

    d. Row totals are inaccurate.

89. Mr. Jones was admitted to the hospital on March 21 and discharged on April 1. What was the length of stay for Mr. Jones?

    a. 5 days

    b. 10 days

    c. 11 days

    d. 15 days

90. Community Hospital discharged nine patients on April 1. The length of stay for each of the patients was as follows: for patient A, 1 day; for patient B, 5 days; for patient C, 3 days; for patient D, 3 days; for patient E, 8 days; for patient F, 8 days; for patient G, 8 days; for patient H, 9 days; patient I, 9 days. What was the median length of stay?

    a. 5 days

    b. 6 days

    c. 8 days

    d. 9 days

91. Community Hospital had 25 inpatient deaths, including newborns, for the month of June. The hospital performed five autopsies for the same period. What was the gross autopsy rate for the hospital for June?

    a. 0.02%

    b. 5%

    c. 20%

    d. 200%

92. If you want to display the parts of a whole in graphic form, what graphic technique would you use?

    a. Table

    b. Histogram

    c. Line graph

    d. Pie chart

93. Which rate describes the probability or risk of illness in a population over a period of time?

    a. Mortality rate

    b. Incidence rate

    c. Morbidity rate

    d. Prevalence rate

94. Which term is used to describe the number of inpatients present at the census-taking time each day plus the number of inpatients who were both admitted and discharged after the census-taking time the previous day?

    a. Inpatient bed occupancy rate

    b. Bed count

    c. Average daily census

    d. Daily inpatient census

95. Which unit of measure is used to indicate the services received by one inpatient in a 24-hour period?

    a. Inpatient service day

    b. Volume of services

    c. Average occupancy charges

    d. Length of stay

96. Which rate is used to compare the number of inpatient deaths to the total number of inpatient deaths and discharges?

    a. Net hospital death rate

    b. Fetal/newborn/maternal hospital death rate

    c. Gross hospital death rate

    d. Adjusted hospital death rate

97. Which term is used to describe the number of calendar days that a patient is hospitalized?

    a. Average length of stay

    b. Length of stay

    c. Occupancy rate

    d. Level of service

98. Which rate compares the number of autopsies performed on hospital inpatients to the total number of inpatient deaths for the same period of time?

    a. Net autopsy rate

    b. Gross autopsy rate

    c. Hospital autopsy rate

    d. Average autopsy rate

99. What term is used for the number of inpatients present at any one time in a healthcare facility?

    a. Average daily census

    b. Census

    c. Inpatient service day

    d. Length of stay

100. What is the official count of inpatients taken at midnight called?

    a. Average daily census

    b. Census

    c. Daily inpatient census

    d. Inpatient service days

101. Which of the following use data from the MDS for long-term care?

    a. Centers for Medicare and Medicaid Services

    b. Home health hospice agencies

    c. Home health agencies

    d. Rehabilitation facilities

102. Which of the following is an internal user of data?

    a. Public health department

    b. State data bank

    c. Hospital administrator

    d. Quality improvement organization

103. Which of the following is a research project in which new treatments and tests are investigated to determine whether they are safe and effective?

    a. Clinical trial

    b. Clinical outcome

    c. Clinical process

    d. Clinical protocol

104. The capture of secondary diagnoses that increase the incidence of CCs and MCCs at final coding may have an impact on:

    a. Query rate

    b. Principal diagnosis

    c. Case mix index

    d. Record review rate

Domain II *Coding*

105. When coding a hydrocystoma of the eyelid, which of the following codes should be used?

216	Benign neoplasm of skin	
	Includes:	
	Blue nevus	
	Dermatofibroma	
	Hydrocystoma	
	Pigmented nevus	
	Syringoadenoma	
	Syringoma	
	Excludes:	
	Skin of genital organs (221.0–222.9)	
216.0	Skin of lip	
	Excludes:	
	Vermilion border of lip (210.0)	
216.1	Eyelid, including canthus	
	Excludes:	
	Cartilage of eyelid (215.0)	

    a. 216

    b. 210.0

    c. 215.0

    d. 216.1

106. When coding a benign neoplasm of skin of the vermilion border of the lip, which of the following codes should be used?

216	Benign neoplasm of skin
	Includes:
	Blue nevus
	Dermatofibroma
	Hydrocystoma
	Pigmented nevus
	Syringoadenoma
	Syringoma
	Excludes:
	Skin of genital organs (221.0–222.9)
216.0	Skin of lip
	Excludes:
	Vermilion border of lip (210.0)
216.2	Eyelid, including canthus
	Excludes:
	Cartilage of eyelid (215.0)

  a. 216

  b. 210.0

  c. 216.0

  d. 216.1

107. If a patient has an excision of a malignant lesion of the skin, the CPT code is determined by the body area from which the excision occurs and which of the following?

  a. Length of the lesion as described in the pathology report

  b. Dimension of the specimen submitted as described in the pathology report

  c. Width times the length of the lesion as described in the operative report

  d. Diameter of the lesion as well as the margins excised as described in the operative report

108. According to CPT, a repair of a laceration that includes retention sutures would be considered what type of closure?

  a. Complex

  b. Intermediate

  c. Not specified

  d. Simple

109. The patient was admitted with nausea, vomiting, and abdominal pain. The physician documents the following on the discharge summary: acute cholecystitis, nausea, vomiting, and abdominal pain. Which of the following would be the correct coding and sequencing for this case?

  a. Acute cholecystitis, nausea, vomiting, abdominal pain

  b. Abdominal pain, vomiting, nausea, acute cholecystitis

  c. Nausea, vomiting, abdominal pain

  d. Acute cholecystitis

110. A patient is admitted with spotting. She had been treated two weeks previously for a miscarriage with sepsis. The sepsis had resolved and she is afebrile at this time. She is treated with an aspiration dilation and curettage. Products of conception are found. Which of the following should be the principal diagnosis?

    a. Miscarriage

    b. Complications of spontaneous abortion with sepsis

    c. Sepsis

    d. Spontaneous abortion with sepsis

111. An 80-year-old female is admitted with fever, lethargy, hypotension, tachycardia, oliguria, and elevated WBC. The patient has more than 100,000 organisms of *Escherichia coli* per cc of urine. The attending physician documents "urosepsis." How should the coder proceed to code this case?

    a. Code sepsis as the principal diagnosis with urinary tract infection due to *E. coli* as secondary diagnosis.

    b. Code urinary tract infection with sepsis as the principal diagnosis.

    c. Query the physician to ask if the patient has septicemia because of the symptomatology.

    d. Query the physician to ask if the patient had septic shock so that this may be used as the principal diagnosis.

112. The practice of using a code that results in a higher payment to the provider than the code that actually reflects the service or item provided is known as:

    a. Unbundling

    b. Upcoding

    c. Medically unnecessary services

    d. Billing for services not provided

113. A 65-year-old patient, with a history of lung cancer, is admitted to a healthcare facility with ataxia and syncope and a fractured arm as a result of falling. The patient undergoes a closed reduction of the fracture in the emergency department and undergoes a complete workup for metastatic carcinoma of the brain. The patient is found to have metastatic carcinoma of the lung to the brain and undergoes radiation therapy to the brain. Which of the following would be the principal diagnosis in this case?

    a. Ataxia

    b. Fractured arm

    c. Metastatic carcinoma of the brain

    d. Carcinoma of the lung

114. A patient was admitted for abdominal pain with diarrhea and was diagnosed with infectious gastroenteritis. The patient also had angina and chronic obstructive pulmonary disease. Which of the following would be the correct coding and sequencing for this case?

    a. Abdominal pain; infectious gastroenteritis; chronic obstructive pulmonary disease; angina

    b. Infectious gastroenteritis; chronic obstructive pulmonary disease; angina

    c. Gastroenteritis; abdominal pain; angina

    d. Gastroenteritis; abdominal pain; diarrhea; chronic obstructive pulmonary disease; angina

115. A patient is admitted with a history of prostate cancer and with mental confusion. The patient completed radiation therapy for prostatic carcinoma three years ago and is status post a radical resection of the prostate. A CT scan of the brain during the current admission reveals metastasis. Which of the following is the correct coding and sequencing for the current hospital stay?

    a. Metastatic carcinoma of the brain; carcinoma of the prostate; mental confusion

    b. Mental confusion; history of carcinoma of the prostate; admission for chemotherapy

    c. Metastatic carcinoma of the brain; history of carcinoma of the prostate

    d. Carcinoma of the prostate; metastatic carcinoma to the brain

116. A patient is admitted with abdominal pain. The physician states that the discharge diagnosis is pancreatitis and noncalculus cholecystitis. Both diagnoses are equally treated. The correct coding and sequencing for this case would be:

    a. Sequence either the pancreatitis or noncalculus cholecystitis as principal diagnosis

    b. Pancreatitis; noncalculus cholecystitis; abdominal pain

    c. Noncalculus cholecystitis; pancreatitis; abdominal pain

    d. Abdominal pain; pancreatitis; noncalculus cholecystitis

117. According to the UHDDS, which of the following is the definition of "other diagnoses"?

    a. Is recorded in the patient record

    b. Is documented by the attending physician and cannot be documented by any other provider

    c. Is considered all conditions that coexist at the time of admission, or develop subsequently, which affect the treatment received and/or the length of stay

    d. Is documented by at least two physicians and/or the nursing staff

118. A 7-year-old patient was admitted to the emergency department for treatment of shortness of breath. The patient is given epinephrine and nebulizer treatments. The shortness of breath and wheezing are unabated following treatment. What diagnosis should be suspected?

    a. Acute bronchitis

    b. Acute bronchitis with chronic obstructive pulmonary disease

    c. Asthma with status asthmaticus

    d. Chronic obstructive asthma

119. A coder might find which of the following on a patient's problem list if the medication list contains the drug Procardia?

    a. Esophagitis

    b. Hypertension

    c. Schizophrenia

    d. AIDS

120. A physician orders a chest x-ray for an office patient who presents with fever, productive cough, and shortness of breath. The physician indicates in the progress notes: "Rule out pneumonia." What should the coder report for the visit when the results have not yet been received?

    a. Pneumonia

    b. Fever, cough, shortness of breath

    c. Cough, shortness of breath

    d. Pneumonia, cough, shortness of breath, fever

121. Given the information here, how much of the APC payment would the facility receive for the status T procedure?

Billing Number	Status Indicator	CPT/HCPCS	APC
998323	V	99285–25	0612
998323	T	25500	0044
998323	X	72050	0261
998323	S	72128	0283
998323	S	70450	0283

    a. 0%

    b. 50%

    c. 75%

    d. 100%

122. Which of the following promotes uniform reporting and statistical data collection for medical procedures, supplies, products, and services?

    a. Current Procedural Terminology

    b. Healthcare Common Procedure Coding System

    c. *International Classification of Diseases, Ninth Revision, Clinical Modification*

    d. *International Classification of Diseases for Oncology,* Third Edition

123. Which of the following provides a detailed classification system for coding the histology, topography, and behavior of neoplasms?

    a. Current Procedural Terminology

    b. Healthcare Common Procedure Coding System

    c. *International Classification of Diseases for Oncology,* Third Edition

    d. Systematized Nomenclature of Medicine Clinical Terminology

124. A 65-year-old woman was admitted to the hospital. She was diagnosed with septicemia secondary to methicillin-susceptible *Staphylococcus aureus* and abdominal pain secondary to diverticulitis of the colon. What is the correct code assignment?

038.11	Methicillin susceptible *Staphylococcus aureus* septicemia
038.8	Other specified septicemia
038.9	Unspecified septicemia
041.11	Methicillin susceptible *Staphylococcus aureus*
562.11	Diverticulitis of colon (without mention of hemorrhage)
789.00	Abdominal pain, unspecified site

   a. 038.8, 562.11, 789.00

   b. 038.11, 562.11

   c. 038.8, 562.11, 041.11

   d. 038.9, 562.11

125. Which of the following provides the most comprehensive controlled vocabulary for coding the content of a patient record?

   a. CPT

   b. HCPCS

   c. ICD-9-CM

   d. SNOMED CT

126. Patient was admitted to the hospital and diagnosed with diabetic gangrene. What is the correct code assignment?

250.00	Diabetes mellitus without mention of complication, type II or unspecified type, not stated as uncontrolled
250.70	Diabetes with peripheral circulatory disorders, type II or unspecified type, not stated as uncontrolled
250.71	Diabetes with peripheral circulatory disorders, type I [juvenile type], not stated as uncontrolled
785.4	Gangrene

   a. 250.71, 785.4

   b. 785.4, 250.70

   c. 250.70, 250.00, 785.4

   d. 250.70, 785.4

127. Which of the following is the planned replacement for ICD-9-CM Volumes 1 and 2?

   a. Current Procedural Terminology (CPT)

   b. *International Classification of Diseases, Tenth Revision, Clinical Modification* (ICD-10-CM and ICD-10-PCS)

   c. *International Classification of Diseases, Tenth Revision* (ICD-10)

   d. *International Classification of Diseases, Tenth Revision, Clinical Modification* (ICD-10-CM)

128. Which organization originally published ICD-9?

    a. American Medical Association

    b. Centers for Disease Control

    c. United States federal government

    d. World Health Organization

129. Which of the following organizations is responsible for updating the procedure classification of ICD-9-CM?

    a. Centers for Disease Control

    b. Centers for Medicare and Medicaid Services

    c. National Center for Health Statistics

    d. World Health Organization

130. At which level of the classification system are the most specific ICD-9-CM codes found?

    a. Category level

    b. Section level

    c. Subcategory level

    d. Subclassification level

131. Assign the correct CPT code for the following procedure: Revision of the pacemaker skin pocket.

    a. 33223, Revision of skin pocket for cardioverter-defibrillator

    b. 33210, Insertion or replacement of temporary transvenous single chamber cardiac electrode or pacemaker catheter (separate procedure)

    c. 33212, Insertion of pacemaker pulse generator only, with existing single lead

    d. 33222, Revision or relocation of skin pocket for pacemaker

132. What are four-digit ICD-9-CM diagnosis codes?

    a. Category codes

    b. Section codes

    c. Subcategory codes

    d. Subclassification codes

133. Assign the correct CPT code for the following: A 63-year-old female had a temporal artery biopsy completed in the outpatient surgical center.

    a. 32405, Biopsy, lung or mediastinum, percutaneous needle

    b. 37609, Ligation or biopsy, temporal artery

    c. 20206, Biopsy, muscle, percutaneous needle

    d. 31629, Bronchoscopy, rigid or flexible, including fluoroscopic guidance, when performed; with transbronchial needle aspiration biopsy(s), trachea, mainstem and/or lobar bronchus(i)

134. Which of the following ICD-9-CM codes classify environmental events and circumstances as the cause of an injury, poisoning, or other adverse effect?

    a. Category codes

    b. E codes

    c. Subcategory codes

    d. V codes

135. A physician query may not be appropriate in which of the following instances?

    a. Diagnosis of viral pneumonia noted in the progress notes and sputum cultures showing *Haemophilus influenzae*

    b. Discharge summary indicates chronic renal failure but the progress notes document acute renal failure throughout the stay

    c. Acute respiratory failure in a patient whose lab report findings appear to not support this diagnosis

    d. Diagnosis of chest pain and abnormal cardiac enzymes indicative of an AMI

136. Which of the following provides a system for coding the clinical procedures and services provided by physicians and other clinical professionals?

    a. Current Procedural Terminology

    b. *Diagnostic and Statistical Manual of Mental Disorders, Fourth Revision*

    c. Healthcare Common Procedure Coding System

    d. *International Classification of Diseases, Ninth Revision, Clinical Modification*

137. Which of the following conditions are included on the hospital-acquired conditions provision list?

    a. Pressure ulcers, *Staphylococcus* infections, gunshot wounds

    b. *Staphylococcus* infections, air embolism, physical and substance abuse

    c. Catheter associated urinary tract infections, gunshot wounds

    d. Pressure ulcers, catheter associated urinary tract infections, falls and fractures

138. The coding manager at Community Hospital is seeing an increased number of physicians failing to document the cause and effect of diabetes and its manifestations. Which of the following will provide the most comprehensive solution to handle this documentation issue?

    a. Have coders continue to query the attending physician for this documentation.

    b. Present this information at the next medical staff meeting to inform physicians on documentation standards and guidelines.

    c. Do nothing because coding compliance guidelines do not allow any action.

    d. Place all offending physicians on suspension if the documentation issues continue.

139. Which of the following elements of coding quality represent the degree to which codes accurately reflect the patient's diagnoses and procedures?

    a. Reliability

    b. Validity

    c. Completeness

    d. Timeliness

140. A patient is admitted to the hospital with acute lower abdominal pain. The principal diagnosis is acute appendicitis. The patient also has a diagnosis of diabetes. The patient undergoes an appendectomy and subsequently develops two wound infections. In the DRG system, which of the following could be considered a comorbid condition?

    a. Acute appendicitis

    b. Appendectomy

    c. Diabetes

    d. Wound infection

141. Given the information here, which of the following statements is correct?

MS-DRG	MDC	Type	MS-DRG Title	Weight	Discharges	Geometric Mean	Arithmetic Mean
191	04	MED	Chronic obstructive pulmonary disease w CC	0.9628	10	3.7	4.5
192	04	MED	Chronic obstructive pulmonary disease w/o CC/MCC	0.7081	20	3.0	3.5
193	04	MED	Simple pneumonia & pleurisy w MCC	1.4948	10	5.2	6.4
194	04	MED	Simple pneumonia & pleurisy w CC	1.0026	20	4.0	4.8
195	04	MED	Simple pneumonia & pleurisy w/o CC/MCC	0.7037	10	3.0	3.6

    a. In each MS-DRG the geometric mean is lower than the arithmetic mean.

    b. In each MS-DRG the arithmetic mean is lower than the geometric mean.

    c. The higher the number of patients in each MS-DRG, the greater the geometric mean for that MS-DRG.

    d. The geometric means are lower in MS-DRGs that are associated with a CC or MCC.

142. Given the following information, in which city is the GPCI the highest for practice expense?

Sample Geographical Practice Cost Indices (GPCI) for Selected Cities			
City	Work GPCI	Practice Expense GPCI	Malpractice Expense GPCI
St. Louis	1.000	0.968	1.064
Dallas	1.009	1.001	0.969
Seattle	1.020	1.098	0.785
Philadelphia	1.015	1.084	1.619

   a. St. Louis

   b. Dallas

   c. Seattle

   d. Philadelphia

143. Given the following information, which of the following has the lowest work RVU?

Sample RVUs for Selected HCPCS Codes				
HCPCS Code	Description	Work RVU	Practice Expense RVU	Malpractice Expense RVU
99204	Office visit	2.43	1.20	0.23
10080	I&D of pilonidal cyst, simple	1.22	1.58	0.20
45380	Colonoscopy with biopsy	4.43	2.72	0.67
52601	TURP, complete	15.26	8.04	1.50

   a. Office visit

   b. I&D of pilonidal cyst, simple

   c. Colonoscopy with biopsy

   d. TURP, complete

144. Which of the following is the condition established after study to be the reason for hospitalization?

   a. Principal procedure

   b. Complication

   c. Comorbidity

   d. Principal diagnosis

145. Which of the following is a prospective payment system implemented for payment of inpatient services?

   a. APC

   b. MS-DRG

   c. OPPS

   d. RBRVS

146. In the inpatient prospective payment system (IPPS), the calculation of the DRG begins with the:

   a. Principal diagnosis

   b. Primary diagnosis

   c. Secondary diagnosis

   d. Surgical procedure

147. Diagnosis-related groups are organized into:

   a. Case-mix classifications

   b. Geographic practice cost indices

   c. Major diagnostic categories

   d. Resource-based relative values

148. NCCI edits prevent improper payments where:

   a. Medical necessity has not been justified by a diagnosis

   b. The account is potentially upcoded

   c. The claim contains any of a variety of errors

   d. Incorrect code combinations are on the claim

149. Medicare inpatient reimbursement levels are based on:

   a. CPT codes reported during the encounter

   b. MS-DRG calculated for the encounter

   c. Charges accumulated during the episode of care

   d. Usual and customary charges reported during the encounter

150. Coding and billing documentation must be based on the:

   a. Wishes of the patient

   b. Highest available reimbursement amount

   c. Most efficient utilization of resources

   d. Provider's documentation

151. Unbundling refers to:

   a. Failure to use a comprehensive code to inappropriately maximize reimbursement

   b. Failure to use multiple procedure codes to inappropriately maximize reimbursement

   c. Combined billing for pre- and post-surgery physician services

   d. Using the incorrect DRG code

152. MS-DRGs may be split into a maximum of _____ payment tiers based on severity as determined by the presence of a major complication/comorbidity, a CC, or no CC.

   a. Two

   b. Three

   c. Four

   d. Five

153. The purpose of the present on admission (POA) indicator is to:

    a. Differentiate between conditions present on admission and conditions that develop during an inpatient admission

    b. Track principal diagnoses

    c. Distinguish between principal and primary diagnoses

    d. Determine principal diagnosis

154. The present on admission (POA) indicator is a requirement for:

    a. Inpatient Medicare claims submitted by hospitals

    b. Inpatient Medicare and Medicaid claims submitted by hospitals

    c. Medicare claims submitted by all entities

    d. Inpatient skilled nursing facility Medicare claims

155. A coding audit shows that an inpatient coder is using multiple codes that describe the individual components of a procedure rather than using a single code that describes all the steps of the procedure performed. Which of the following should be done in this case?

    a. Require all coders to implement this practice

    b. Report the practice to the OIG

    c. Counsel the coder and stop the practice immediately

    d. Put the coder on unpaid leave of absence

156. The National Correct Coding Initiative (NCCI) was developed to control improper coding leading to inappropriate payment for:

    a. Part A Medicare claims

    b. Part B Medicare claims

    c. Medicaid claims

    d. Medicare and Medicaid claims

157. The function of the NCCI editor is to:

    a. Report poor performing physicians

    b. Identify procedures and services that cannot be billed together on the same day of service for a patient.

    c. Identify poor performing coders

    d. Identify problems in the national coding system

158. NCCI edit files contain code pairs called mutually exclusive edits, which prevent payment for:

    a. Services that cannot reasonably be billed together

    b. Services that are components of a more comprehensive procedure

    c. Unnecessary procedures

    d. Comprehensive procedures

159. The evaluation of coders is recommended at least quarterly for the purpose of measurement and assurance of:

    a. Speed

    b. Data quality and integrity

    c. Accuracy

    d. Effective relationships with physicians and facility personnel

160. Quality standards for coding accuracy should be:

    a. At least 90%

    b. At least 95%

    c. As close to 100% as possible

    d. No specific standards are possible

161. The acute-care hospital discharges an average of 55 patients per day. The HIM department is open during normal business hours only. The volume productivity standard is six records per hour when coding 4.5 hours per day. Assuming that standards are met, how many FTE coders does the facility need to have on staff in order to ensure that there is no backlog?

    a. 2.85

    b. 5

    c. 14.26

    d. 27

162. A coder notes that the patient is taking prescribed Haldol. The final diagnoses on the progress notes include diabetes mellitus, acute pharyngitis, and malnutrition. What condition might the coder suspect the patient has and should query the physician?

    a. Insomnia

    b. Hypertension

    c. Mental or behavior problems

    d. Rheumatoid arthritis

163. Mary Patient presented to the emergency department with chest pains and shortness of breath. She was treated for congestive heart failure and returned home. Two days later, her symptoms had worsened. She presented again to the emergency department and was admitted to the hospital for inpatient treatment of congestive heart failure. The hospital will bill Medicare for:

    a. Two emergency department visits as an outpatient service and the inpatient visit under MS-DRGs

    b. One inpatient visit under MS-DRGs

    c. One emergency department visit as an outpatient service and one inpatient visit under MS-DRGs

    d. Two emergency department visits as an outpatient service and the inpatient visit at a reduced rate under MS-DRGs

164. The coding supervisor has compiled a report on the number of coding errors made each day by the coding staff. The report data show that Tim makes an average of six errors per day, Jane makes an average of five errors per day, and Bob and Susan each make an average of two errors per day. Given this information, what action should the coding supervisor take?

    a. Counsel Tim and Jane because they have the highest error rates.

    b. Encourage Tim and Jane to get additional training.

    c. Provide Bob and Susan with incentive pay for low coding error rate.

    d. Take no action since not enough information is given to make a judgment.

165. The patient was admitted to the outpatient department and had a bronchoscopy with bronchial brushings performed.

31622	Bronchoscopy, rigid or flexible, including fluoroscopic guidance, when performed, diagnostic, with cell washing when performed (separate procedure)
31023	Bronchoscopy, rigid or flexible, including fluoroscopic guidance, when performed; with brushing or protected brushings
31625	Bronchoscopy, rigid or flexible, including fluoroscopic guidance, when performed; with bronchial or endobronchial biopsy(s), single or multiple sites
31640	Bronchoscopy, rigid or flexible, including fluoroscopic guidance, when performed; with excision of tumor

    a. 31622, 31640

    b. 31622, 31623

    c. 31623

    d. 31625

166. The practice of undercoding can affect a hospital's MS-DRG case mix in which of the following ways?

    a. Makes it lower than warranted by the actual service/resource intensity of the facility.

    b. Makes it higher than warranted by the actual service/resource intensity of the facility.

    c. Does not affect the hospital's MS-DRG case mix.

    d. Coding has nothing to do with a hospital's MS-DRG case mix.

167. Which condition is not included on the hospital-acquired conditions provision list for FY 2009?

    a. Pressure ulcers

    b. *Staphylococcus* infections

    c. Catheter associated urinary tract infections

    d. Air embolism

168. When multiple burns are present, the first sequenced diagnosis is the:

    a. Burn that is treated surgically

    b. Burn that is closest to the head

    c. Highest-degree burn

    d. Burn that is treated first

169. A coding professional may assume a cause-and-effect relationship between hypertension and which of the following complications?

    a. Hypertension and heart disease

    b. Hypertension and chronic kidney disease

    c. Hypertension and heart and chronic kidney disease

    d. Hypertension and coronary artery disease

170. A patient with known AIDS is admitted to the hospital for treatment of *Pneumocystis carinii* pneumonia. Assign the principal diagnosis for this patient:

    a. 042, Human immunodeficiency virus [HIV disease]

    b. 486, Pneumonia, organism unspecified

    c. 136.3, Pneumocystosis due to *Pneumocystis carinii*

    d. V08, Asymptomatic human immunodeficiency virus [HIV] infection

171. Coding productivity is measured by:

    a. Quantity

    b. Quality

    c. Quantity and quality

    d. Volume

172. The _____ is responsible for issuing official coding guidelines for ICD-9-CM, whereas the _____ is responsible for issuing official guidelines for CPT.

    a. AHIMA, AMA

    b. AMA, AHA

    c. AHIMA, AMA

    d. AHA, AMA

173. Medicare outpatients are grouped by:

    a. APC

    b. PPS

    c. DRG

    d. CMS

174. Which of the following could be a focus of a quality review program?

    a. CC and MCC coding rates (MS-DRGs)

    b. Outpatient Code Editor failure rates

    c. Coding completed by new coders

    d. New coding guidelines

175. Which of the following is *not* a reason for establishing a coding quality program?

    a. Proactively identify variations in coding practices among staff members

    b. Determine the cause and scope of identified problems

    c. Identify which coder should be disciplined

    d. Set priorities for resolving identified problems

176. What is the benefit to comparing the coding assigned by coders to the coding appearing on the claim?

    a. May find that more codes are required to support the claim

    b. May find that the charge description master soft coding is inaccurate

    c. Serves as a way for HIM to take over the management of patient financial services

    d. Could find claim generation issues that cannot be found other ways

177. MCC stands for:

    a. Massive complication/comorbid condition

    b. Many chronic conditions

    c. Much chronic congestion

    d. Major complication and comorbidity

178. A patient in seen as an outpatient to receive radiation and chemotherapy for distal esophageal carcinoma. What is the appropriate first-listed diagnosis?

    a. V58.42, Aftercare following surgery for a neoplasm

    b. V58.11, Encounter for antineoplastic chemotherapy

    c. 150.5, Malignant neoplasm of esophagus, lower third of esophagus

    d. 150.3, Malignant neoplasm of esophagus, upper third of esophagus

179. When the physician does not specify the method used to remove a lesion during an endoscopy, what is the appropriate procedure?

    a. Assign the removal by snare technique code

    b. Assign the removal by hot biopsy forceps code

    c. Assign the ablation code

    d. Query the physician as to the method used

180. A 30-year-old female has a vaginal delivery with single liveborn female with episiotomy and repair.

650	Normal delivery
664.41	Unspecified perineal laceration, delivered, with or without mention of antepartum condition
665.40	High-vaginal laceration, unspecified as to episode of care or not applicable
V27.0	Single liveborn
73.6	Episiotomy (with subsequent repair)
75.69	Repair of other current obstetric laceration

    a. 664.41, V27.0, 73.6, 75.69

    b. 650, V27.0, 73.6; 75.69

    c. 650, V27.0, 73.6

    d. 665.40, 73.6

181. The hospital-acquired conditions provision of the Medicare PPS is an example of this type of value-based purchasing system?

    a. Paying for value

    b. Penalty-based

    c. Reward-based

    d. Penalty for value

182. Which of the following procedures or services could *not* be assigned a code with CPT?

    a. Gastroscopy

    b. Anesthesia

    c. Glucose tolerance test

    d. Crutches

183. Which of the following would be classified in ICD-9-CM with an E code?

    a. Echocardiogram

    b. Fall from curb

    c. Adenocarcinoma

    d. Admission for plastic surgery

184. The physician documents that she changed the cardiac pacemaker battery. In CPT, the battery is called a(n):

    a. Generator

    b. Electrode

    c. Dual system

    d. Cardioverter

185. A patient is scheduled for an outpatient colonoscopy, but due to a sudden drop in blood pressure, the procedure is cancelled just as the scope is introduced into the rectum. Because of moderately severe mental retardation, the patient is given general anesthetic prior to the procedure. How should this procedure be coded?

    a. Assign the code for colonoscopy with modifier –74, Discontinued outpatient procedure after anesthesia administration

    b. Assign the code for a colonoscopy with modifier –52, Reduced services

    c. Assign no code because no procedure was performed

    d. Assign an anesthesia code only

186. When documentation in the health record is not clear, the coding professional should:

    a. Submit the question to coding clinic

    b. Refer to dictation from other encounters for the patient to get clarification

    c. Query the physician who originated the progress note or other report in question

    d. Query a physician who consistently responds to queries in a timely manner

187. Providers should be queried regarding information in the health record for all of the following *except*:

    a. Conflicting documentation

    b. Ambiguous documentation

    c. Incomplete information

    d. Insignificant information

188. MS-DRG refers to a DRG system developed by:

    a. Microsoft

    b. 3M Corporation

    c. Yale University

    d. CMS

189. The _____ operates in the systems of Medicare administrative contractors (MACs) and provides a series of flags that can affect APC payments because it identifies coding errors in claims.

    a. POA

    b. OCE

    c. CPT

    d. DRG

190. The main purpose of Correct Coding Initiative (CCI) edits is to prohibit:

    a. ICD-9-CM procedure code errors

    b. DRG assignment errors

    c. Unbundling of procedures

    d. Incorrect POA assignment

191. Continuing education is vital to ensure accurate coding. All of the following are true about continuing education for coders *except*:

    a. Physicians from the medical staff can be asked to present clinical topics to coders

    b. Coding managers can use member resources from AHIMA to educate coders

    c. Coding education is best accomplished by sending staff to external seminars

    d. Coding managers can have coders research clinical topics to present to each other

192. Which of the following would generally be found in a query to a physician?

    a. Health record number and demographic information

    b. Name and contact number of the individual initiating the query and account number

    c. Date query initiated and date query must be completed

    d. Demographic information and name and contact number of individual initiating the query

193. An accuracy calculation method that divides the number of records where there was no change in APC or DRG assignment by the total number of cases reviewed is considered:

    a. Code over code method

    b. Record over record method

    c. Code over record method

    d. Code determination method

194. An outcome of coding quality reviews may be any of the following, *except*:

    a. Coding documentation issues that prevent the coders from performing comprehensive coding are identified

    b. Redundant codes on the claims are identified

    c. Cases where excellent penmanship created challenges for the coders are identified

    d. Areas where coding could be improved if a physician was queried are identified

195. When assigning evaluation and management codes for hospital outpatient services, the coder should follow:

    a. AHA guidelines

    b. AHIMA guidelines

    c. CMS guidelines

    d. The hospital's own internal guidelines

196. Which of the following is *not* one of the components that make up the total relative value unit (RVU) for a given procedure?

    a. Staff work

    b. Physician work

    c. Practice expense

    d. Malpractice expense

197. Which of the following neoplasm types is correct for adenocarcinoma?

    a. Benign

    b. Malignant

    c. Uncertain behavior

    d. Unspecified

Domain III *Compliance* Start: 5:22 End: 6:10 (was watching t.v.)

198. OASIS data are used to assess the _____ of home health services.

    a. Outcome

    b. Financial performance

    c. Utilization

    d. Core measure

199. A statement or guideline that directs decision making or behavior is called a:

a. Directive

b. Procedure

c. Policy

d. Process

200. Examples of high-risk billing practices that create compliance risks for healthcare organizations include all of the following, *except*:

a. Altered claim forms

b. Returned overpayments

c. Duplicate billings

d. Unbundled procedures

201. Healthcare fraud is all of the following *except*:

a. Unnecessary costs to a program

b. False representation of fact

c. Failure to disclose a material fact

d. Damage to another party that reasonably relied on misrepresentation

202. Corporate compliance programs became common after adoption of which of the following:

a. False Claims Act

b. Federal Sentencing Guidelines

c. Office of the Inspector General for HHS

d. Federal Physician Self-Referral Statute

203. Which of the following is a legal concern regarding the EHR?

a. Ability to subpoena audit trails

b. Template design

c. ANSI standards

d. Data sets

204. The act of granting approval to a healthcare organization based on whether the organization has met a set of voluntary standards is called:

a. Accreditation

b. Licensure

c. Acceptance

d. Approval

205. A group practice has hired an HIT as its chief compliance officer. The current compliance program includes written standards of conduct and policies and procedures that address specific areas of potential fraud. It also has audits in place to monitor compliance. Which of the following should the compliance officer also ensure are in place?

    a. Compliance program education and training programs for all employees in the organization

    b. A hotline to receive complaints and adoption of procedures to protect whistleblowers from retaliation

    c. Procedures to adequately identify individuals who make complaints so that appropriate follow-up can be conducted

    d. A corporate compliance committee that reports directly to the CFO

206. In developing a coding compliance program, which of the following would *not* be ordinarily included as participants in coding compliance education?

    a. Current coding personnel

    b. Medical staff

    c. Newly hired coding personnel

    d. Nursing staff

207. Which of the following organizations within the federal government is responsible for looking at the issues related to the efficiency and effectiveness of the healthcare delivery system, disease protocols, and guidelines for improved disease outcomes?

    a. Agency for Healthcare Research and Quality (AHRQ)

    b. Food and Drug Administration (FDA)

    c. National Center for Health Statistics (NCHS)

    d. Centers for Medicare and Medicaid Services (CMS)

208. Which of the following issues compliance program guidance?

    a. AHIMA

    b. CMS

    c. *Federal Register*

    d. HHS Office of Inspector General (OIG)

209. Which of the following is an example of data security?

    a. Automatic logoff after inactivity

    b. Fire protection

    c. Contingency planning

    d. Card key for access to data center

210. A patient has been discharged prior to an administrative utilization review being conducted. Which of the following should be performed?

    a. Continued stay utilization review

    b. Discharge plan

    c. Retrospective utilization review

    d. Case management

211. An EHR system can provide better security than a paper record for protected health information system due to:

    a. Handling by fewer clinical practitioners

    b. Access controls, audit trails, and authentication systems

    c. Easier data entry

    d. Safer storage

212. Community Hospital wants to provide transcription services for transcription of office notes of the private patients of physicians. All of these physicians have medical staff privileges at the hospital. This will provide an essential service to the physicians as well as provide additional revenue for the hospital. In preparing to launch this service, the HIM director is asked whether a business associate agreement is necessary. Which of the following should the hospital HIM director advise to comply with HIPAA regulations?

    a. Each physician practice should obtain a business associate agreement with the hospital.

    b. The hospital should obtain a business associate agreement with each physician practice.

    c. Because the physicians all have medical staff privileges, no business associate agreement is necessary.

    d. Because the physicians are part of an Organized Health Care Arrangement (OHCA) with the hospital, no business associate agreement is necessary.

213. Which accrediting organization has instituted continuous improvement and sentinel event monitoring and uses tracer methodology during survey visits?

    a. Accreditation Association for Ambulatory Healthcare

    b. Commission on Accreditation of Rehabilitation Facilities

    c. American Osteopathic Association

    d. The Joint Commission

214. Developing, implementing, and revising the organization's policies is the role of:

    a. Senior managers

    b. The Board of Directors

    c. Supervisory managers

    d. Middle managers

215. Position descriptions, policies and procedures, training checklists, and performance standards are all examples of:

    a. Staffing tools

    b. Organizational policies

    c. Strategic plans

    d. Items on a training checklist

216. This organization has been responsible for accrediting healthcare organizations since the mid 1950s and determines whether the organization is continually monitoring and improving the quality of care they provide.

    a. Commission on Accreditation of Rehabilitation Facilities

    b. American Osteopathic Association

    c. National Committee for Quality Assurance

    d. The Joint Commission

217. Which of the following is a written description of an organization's formal position?

    a. Hierarchy chart

    b. Organizational chart

    c. Policy

    d. Procedure

218. The Deficit Reduction Act of 2005:

    a. Encouraged voluntary compliance programs

    b. Did not address healthcare fraud and abuse

    c. Made compliance programs mandatory

    d. Affects entities that make or receive at least $9 million in Medicaid payments

219. Which of the following statements best defines utilization management?

    a. It is the process of determining whether the medical care provided to a patient is necessary.

    b. It is a set of processes used to determine the appropriateness of medical services provided during specific episodes of care.

    c. It is a process that determines whether a planned service or a patient's condition warrants care in an inpatient setting.

    d. It is an ongoing infection surveillance program.

220. Which of the following is *not* a type of utilization review?

    a. Preadmission review

    b. Continued-stay review

    c. Discharge review

    d. Peer review

221. Which of the following is *not* one of the basic functions of the utilization review process?

    a. Case management

    b. Discharge planning

    c. Claims management

    d. Utilization review

222. The Medical Record Committee wants to determine if the hospital is in compliance with Joint Commission standards for medical record delinquency rates. The HIM director has compiled a report that shows that records are delinquent for an average of 29 days after discharge. Given this information, what can the Committee conclude?

    a. Delinquency rate is within Joint Commission standards.

    b. All physicians are performing at optimal levels.

    c. The chart deficiency process is working well.

    d. Data are insufficient to determine whether the hospital is in compliance.

223. Which of the following is the largest healthcare standards-setting body in the world?

    a. Agency for Healthcare Research and Quality

    b. National Guideline Clearinghouse

    c. National Committee for Quality Assurance

    d. The Joint Commission

224. Community Hospital wants to offer information technology services to City Hospital, another smaller hospital in the area. This arrangement will financially help both institutions. In reviewing the process to establish this arrangement, the CEO asks the HIM director if there are any barriers to establishing this relationship with regard to HIPAA. In this situation, which of the following should the HIM director advise?

    a. There are no barriers prescribed by HIPAA for this arrangement.

    b. Community Hospital needs to expand their organized healthcare arrangement to include the other hospital.

    c. City Hospital should obtain a business associate agreement with Community Hospital.

    d. Community Hospital should obtain a business associate agreement with City Hospital.

225. Which of the following facilities do *not* have to meet the standards in the Conditions of Participation?

    a. Hospitals

    b. Physician offices

    c. Home health agencies

    d. Hospices

226. An audit trail may be used to detect which of the following:

    a. Unauthorized access to a system

    b. Loss of data

    c. Presence of a virus

    d. Successful completion of a backup

227. Specific performance expectations and/or structures and processes that provide detailed information for each of the Joint Commission standards are called:

    a. Elements of performance

    b. Fact sheets

    c. Ad hoc reports

    d. Registers

228. The creation of the National Practitioner Data Bank was mandated by the:

    a. Social Security Act

    b. Privacy Act

    c. Health Insurance Portability and Accountability Act (HIPAA)

    d. Health Care Quality Improvement Act

229. Which of the following dictates how the medical staff operates?

    a. Medical staff classification

    b. Medical staff bylaws

    c. Medical staff credentialing

    d. Medical staff committees

230. Who is responsible for implementing the policies and strategic direction of the hospital or healthcare organization and for building an effective executive management team?

    a. Board of Directors

    b. Chief executive officer

    c. Chief information officer

    d. Chief of staff

231. Medical school graduates must pass a test before they can obtain a _____ to practice medicine.

    a. Degree

    b. Residency

    c. Specialty

    d. License

232. Under HIPAA rules, when an individual asks to see his or her own health information, a covered entity:

    a. Must always provide access

    b. Can deny access to psychotherapy notes

    c. Can demand that the individual pay to see his or her record

    d. Can always deny access

233. In which of the following situations must a covered entity provide an appeals process for denials to requests from individuals to see their own health information?

    a. When access to psychotherapy notes is requested

    b. When the covered entity is a correctional institution

    c. When a licensed healthcare professional has determined that access to PHI would likely endanger the life or safety of the individual

    d. When the covered entity has acted under the direction of a correctional institution

234. Which of the following statements is true in regard to responding to requests from individuals for access to their PHI?

    a. A cost-based fee may be charged for retrieval of the PHI.

    b. A cost-based fee may be charged for making a copy of the PHI.

    c. No fees of any type may be charged.

    d. A minimal fee may be charged for retrieval and copying of PHI.

235. Which of the following is *not* an automatic control that helps preserve data confidentiality and integrity in an electronic system?

    a. Edit checks

    b. Audit trails

    c. Password management

    d. Security awareness program

236. Within the context of data security, protecting data privacy means defending or safeguarding:

    a. Access to information

    b. Data availability

    c. Health record quality

    d. System implementation

237. The protection measures and tools for safeguarding information and information systems is a definition of:

    a. Confidentiality

    b. Data security

    c. Informational privacy

    d. Informational access control

238. To date the HIM department has not charged for copies of records requested by the patient. However, the policy is currently under review for revision. One HIM committee member suggests using the copying fee established by the state. Another committee member thinks that HIPAA will not allow for copying fees. What input should the HIM director provide?

    a. HIPAA does not allow charges for copying of medical records.

    b. Use the state formula because HIPAA allows hospitals to use the state formula.

    c. Base charges on the cost of labor and supplies for copying and postage if copies are mailed.

    d. Because HIPAA restricts charges to the cost of paper, charge only for the paper used for copying the records.

239. A risk analysis is useful to:

    a. Identify security threats

    b. Identify which employees should have access to data

    c. Establish password controls

    d. Establish audit controls

240. Which of the following is required by HIPAA standards?

    a. A written contingency plan

    b. Review of audit trails every 24 hours

    c. Use of passwords for all transactions

    d. Permanent bolting of workstations in public areas

241. Which of the following are policies and procedures required by HIPAA that address the management of computer resources and security?

    a. Access controls

    b. Administrative safeguards

    c. Audit safeguards

    d. Role-based controls

242. What is the biggest threat to the security of healthcare data?

    a. Natural disasters

    b. Fires

    c. Employees

    d. Equipment malfunctions

243. To ensure relevancy, an organization's security policies and procedures be reviewed at least:

    a. Once every six months

    b. Once a year

    c. Every two years

    d. Every five years

244. Which of the following is *not* true of good electronic forms design?

    a. Minimize keystrokes by using pop-up menus.

    b. Perform completeness check for all required data.

    c. Use radio buttons to select multiple items from a set of options.

    d. Use text boxes to enter text.

245. What committee usually oversees the development and approval of new forms for the health record?

    a. Quality review committee

    b. Medical staff committee

    c. Executive committee

    d. Clinical forms committee

246. The process of determining whether the medical care provided to a specific patient is necessary according to preestablished objective screening criteria is:

    a. Activities of daily living assessment

    b. Case management

    c. Patient advocacy

    d. Utilization review

247. Placing locks on computer room doors is considered what type of security control?

    a. Access control

    b. Workstation control

    c. Physical control

    d. Security breach

248. Which of the following is recommended for design of forms for an EDMS?

    a. 24 lb. paper for double-sided forms

    b. 12 lb. paper for double-sided forms

    c. Color-coded paper to make identification easy

    d. 10-digit bar code for identification of each document

249. The HIM supervisor suspects that a departmental employee is accessing the EHR for personal reasons but has no specific data to support this suspicion. In this case, what should the supervisor do?

    a. Confront the employee.

    b. Send out a memorandum to all department employees reminding them of the hospital policy on Internet use.

    c. Ask the security officer for audit trail data to confirm or disprove the suspicion.

    d. Transfer the employee to another job that does not require computer usage.

250. Coding policies should include which of the following elements?

    a. Lunch/break schedule

    b. How to access the computer system

    c. AHIMA Standards of Ethical Coding

    d. Nonofficial coding guidelines

251. The Medicare Integrity Program was established as part of Title II of HIPAA to battle fraud and abuse and is charged with which of the following responsibilities?

    a. Audit of expense reports and notifying beneficiaries of their rights

    b. Payment determinations and audit of cost reports

    c. Publishing of new coding guidelines and code changes

    d. Monitoring of physician credentials and payment determinations

252. An individual designated as an inpatient coder may have access to an electronic medical record to code the record. Under what access security mechanism is the coder allowed access to the system?

    a. Role-based

    b. User-based

    c. Context-based

    d. Situation-based

253. A secretary in the Nursing Office was recently hospitalized with ketoacidosis. She comes to the health information management department and requests to review her health record. Of the options here, what is the best course of action?

    ⌄a. Allow her to review her record after obtaining authorization from her.

    b. Refer the patient to her physician for the information.

    c. Tell her to go through her supervisor for the information.

    d. Tell her that hospital employees cannot access their own medical records

254. St. Joseph's Hospital has a psychiatric service on the sixth floor of the hospital. A 31-year-old male has come to the HIM department and requested to see a copy of his medical record. He indicated he was a patient of Dr. Schmidt, a psychiatrist, and that he was on the sixth floor of St. Joseph's for the last two months. These records are not psychotherapy notes. Of the options here, what is the best course of action?

    a. Prohibit the patient from accessing his record, as it contains psychiatric diagnoses that may greatly upset him.

    b. Allow the patient to access his record.

    c. Allow the patient to access his record if, after contacting his physician, his physician does not think it will be harmful to the patient.

    d. Deny access because HIPAA prevents patients from reviewing their psychiatric records.

255. Minors are basically deemed legally incompetent to access, use, or disclose their health information. What resource should be consulted in terms of who may authorize access, use, or disclose the health records of minors?

    a. HIPAA because there are strict HIPAA rules regarding minors.

    b. Hospital attorneys because they know the rules of the hospital.

    c. State law because HIPAA defers to state laws on matters related to minors.

    d. Federal law because HIPAA overrides state laws on matters related to minors.

256. If an HIM department acts in deliberate ignorance or in disregard of official coding guideline, it may be committing:

    a. Abuse

    b. Fraud

    c. Malpractice

    d. Kickbacks

257. What is the general name for Medicare rules affecting healthcare organizations?

    a. Conditions of Participation

    b. Regulations for Licensure

    c. Requirements for Service

    d. Terms of Accreditation

258. The permanent RAC program was completely implemented in the United States by:

   a. January 2010

   b. March 2011

   c. December 2009

   d. October 2012

259. During user acceptance testing of a new EHR system, physicians are complaining that they have to use multiple log-on screens to access all the system modules. For example, they have to use one log-on for CPOE and another log-on to view laboratory results. One physician suggests having a single sign-on that would provide access to all the EHR system components. However, the hospital administrator thinks that one log-on would be a security issue. What information should the HIM director provide?

   a. Single sign-on is not supported by HIPAA security measures

   b. Single sign-on is discouraged by the Joint Commission

   c. Single sign-on is less frustrating for the end user and can provide better security

   d. Single sign-on is not possible given today's technology

260. Which of the following are security safeguards that protect equipment, media, and facilities?

   a. Administrative controls

   b. Audit controls

   c. Physical access controls

   d. Role based controls

261. What does the term *access control* mean?

   a. Identifying the greatest security risks

   b. Identifying which data employees should have a right to use

   c. Implementing safeguards that protect physical media

   d. Restricting access to computer rooms and facilities

262. Which of the following is a software program that tracks every access to data in the computer system?

   a. Access control

   b. Audit trail

   c. Edit check

   d. Risk assessment

263. All of the following are steps in medical necessity and utilization review, *except*:

   a. Initial clinical review

   b. Peer clinical review

   c. Access consideration

   d. Appeals consideration

264. Which of the following can be used to discover current hot areas of compliance?

    a. The OIG workplan

    b. AHA newsletter

    c. HIPAA Privacy Rule

    d. Local medical review policy

265. In Medicare, the most common forms of fraud and abuse include all of the following *except*:

    a. Billing for services not furnished

    b. Misrepresenting the diagnosis to justify payment

    c. Unbundling or exploding charges

    d. Implementing a clinical documentation improvement program

266. The one aspect of managed care that has had the greatest impact on healthcare organizations is:

    a. Infection control

    b. Cost control

    c. Risk management

    d. Utilization management

267. The policies and procedures section of a coding compliance plan should include all of the following *except*:

    a. Physician query process

    b. Unbundling

    c. Assignment of discharge destination codes

    d. Utilization review

268. What is the term for an explicit statement that directs clinical decision making?

    a. Cookbook medicine

    b. Preauthorization

    c. Evidence-based practice guideline

    d. Withhold pool

269. Gatekeepers determine the appropriateness of all of the following components *except*:

    a. Rate of capitation or reimbursement

    b. Healthcare service itself

    c. Level of healthcare personnel

    d. Setting in the continuum of care

270. Exceptions to the Federal Anti-Kickback Statute that allow legitimate business arrangements and are not subject to prosecution are:

    a. Qui tam practices

    b. Safe practices

    c. Safe harbors

    d. Exclusions

271. How often are healthcare facilities required to practice their emergency preparedness plan annually?

    a. Once

    , b. Twice

    c. Three times

    d. Never

272. This private, not-for-profit organization is committed to developing and maintaining practical, customer-focused standards to help organizations measure and improve the quality, value, and outcomes of behavioral health and medical rehabilitation programs.

    a. Commission on Accreditation of Rehabilitation Facilities

    b. American Osteopathic Association

    c. National Committee for Quality Assurance

    d. The Joint Commission

273. What is it called when accrediting bodies such as The Joint Commission can survey facilities for compliance with the Medicare Conditions of Participation for Hospitals instead of the government?

    a. Deemed status

    b. Judicial decision

    c. Subpoena

    d. Credentialing

274. Which Joint Commission survey methodology involves an evaluation that follows the hospital experiences of past or current patients?

    a. Priority focus process review

    b. Periodic performance review

    c. Tracer methodology

    d. Performance improvement

275. Which of the following services is most likely to be considered medically necessary?

    a. Caregivers' convenience or relief

    b. Cosmetic improvement

    c. Investigational cancer prevention

    d. Standard of care for health condition

276. Case management coordinates an individual's care, especially in complex and high cost cases. Goals of case management include all of the following *except*:

    a. Continuity of care

    b. Quality

    c. Information security

    d. Appropriate utilization

277. When a service is not considered medically necessary based on the reason for encounter, the patient should be provided with a(n) _____ indicating that Medicare might not pay and that the patient might be responsible for the entire charge.

    a. OIG

    b. ABN

    c. LOS

    d. EOB

Domain IV   *Information Technology*

Start: 8:45pm End: 9:50pm (watching t.v)

278. The number that has been proposed for use as a unique patient identification number but is controversial because of confidentiality and privacy concerns is the:

    a. Social security number

    b. Unique physician identification number

    c. Health record number

    d. National provider identifier

279. HIM professionals have been working with a multidisciplinary committee to identify the best solution that will allow hospital physicians coordinated access to all forms of incoming and outgoing messages including voice, fax, e-mail, and video mail. Currently, physicians have to log in to various systems, using different IDs and passwords to retrieve all their messages, reducing effectiveness and efficiency. Which of the following would provide the best solution to the current problem?

    a. Computer–telephone integration (CTI)

    b. Kiosk

    c. IP telephony

    d. Unified messaging

280. The chief information officer is a senior-level executive who is responsible for:

    a. Managing the security of all patient-identifiable information

    b. Ensuring the organization's compliance with federal and state governments and accrediting body rules and regulations on confidentiality

    c. Ensuring the IS implementation plans are in line with the organization's strategic vision

    d. Leading the organizations strategic IS planning process

281. Which of the following is *not* a true statement about a hybrid health record system?

    a. Development of processes for both manual and computer processes is a challenge.

    b. Creation of a definition of what constitutes a health record in manual and electronic format must be developed.

    c. Version control is easy to implement.

    d. Security safeguards must be developed for both paper and electronic processes.

282. Which of the following would be the best course of action to take to ensure continuous availability of electronic data?

    a. Acquire storage management software

    b. Send data to a remote site via the Internet

    c. Store data on RAID

    d. Use mirrored processing on redundant servers

283. Which of the following technologies would allow a hospital to get as much medical record information online as quickly as possible?

    a. Clinical data repository

    b. Picture archiving system

    c. Electronic document management system

    d. Speech recognition system

284. Which of the following technologies would be best for a hospital to use to manage data from its laboratory, pharmacy, and radiology information systems?

    a. Electronic document management system

    b. Clinical data repository

    c. Picture archival system

    d. COLD system

285. Which of the following is necessary to ensure that each term used in an EHR has a common meaning to all users?

    a. Encoded vocabulary

    b. Controlled vocabulary

    c. Data exchange standards

    d. Proprietary standards

286. Why does an ideal EHR system require point-of-care charting?

    a. Eases duplicate data entry burden

    b. Eliminates intermediary paper forms

    c. Reduces memory loss

    d. Ensures that appropriate data are collected

287. Which of the following is a transition strategy to achieve an EHR?

    a. Ancillary system support

    b. Clinical data repository

    c. Electronic document management system

    d. Results retrieval

288. To ensure that a computerized provider order entry (CPOE) system supports patient safety, what other system must also be in place?

    a. Digital dictation

    b. Electronic nursing notes

    c. Pharmacy information system

    d. Point of care charting

289. Which of the following is the unique identifier in the relational database patient table?

Patient Table			
Patient #	Patient Last Name	Patient First Name	Date of Birth
021234	Smith	Donna	03/21/1944
022366	Jones	Donna	04/09/1960
034457	Smith	Mary	08/21/1977

    a. Patient last name

    b. Patient last and first name

    c. Patient date of birth

    d. Patient number

290. As part of an EHR system selection, due diligence should be done:

    a. After installing an EHR to test for acceptance

    b. Before contracting for an EHR product

    c. During system build to check interface quality

    d. Prior to any user authorization for access to data

291. Which of the following tasks is *not* performed in an electronic health record system?

    a. Document imaging

    b. Analysis

    c. Assembly

    d. Indexing

292. A step-by-step approach to installing, testing, training, and gaining adoption for an EHR is referred to as:

    a. Implementation plan

    b. Migration path

    c. Readiness assessment

    d. Strategic plan

293. Which of the following is an application that uses standard order sets and other clinical decision support that supports physician order entry into the computer?

a. CPOE

b. EHR

c. PDA

d. RHIO

294. Electronic systems used by nurses and physicians to document assessments and findings are called:

a. Computerized provider order entry

b. Electronic document management systems

c. Electronic medication administration record

d. Electronic point-of-care charting

295. In the relational database shown here, the patient table and the visit table are related by:

Patient Table			
Patient #	Patient Last Name	Patient First Name	Date of Birth
021234	Smith	Donna	03/21/1944
022366	Jones	William	04/09/1960
034457	Collins	Mary	08/21/1977

Visit Table			
Visit #	Date of Visit	Practitioner #	Patient #
0045678	11/12/2008	456	021234
0045679	11/12/2008	997	021234
0045680	11/12/2008	456	034457

a. Visit number

b. Date of visit

c. Patient number

d. Practitioner number

296. A key element in effective systems implementation is:

a. Contract negotiation

b. User training

c. System evaluation

d. RFP analysis

297. The director of health information services is allowed access to the medical record tracking system when providing the proper log-in and password. Under what access security mechanism is the director allowed access to the system?

    a. Role-based

    b. User-based

    c. Context-based

    d. Situation-based

298. A special web page that offers secure access to data is a(n):

    a. Internet

    b. Home page

    c. Intranet

    d. Portal

299. When some computers are used primarily to enter data and others to process data the architecture is called:

    a. Client/server

    b. Local area network (LAN)

    c. Mainframe

    d. Web services

300. The ability to electronically send data from one electronic system to a different electronic system and still retain its meaning is called:

    a. Data comparability

    b. National data exchange

    c. Interoperability

    d. Data architecture

301. To effectively transmit healthcare data between a provider and payer, both parties must adhere to which electronic data interchange standard?

    a. X12N

    b. LOINC

    c. IEEE 1073

    d. DICOM

302. Who are the primary users of the health record for delivery of healthcare services?

    a. Clinical professionals who provide direct patient care

    b. Insurance companies that cover healthcare expenses

    c. Billers in the healthcare facility's business office

    d. Patients and their families

303. The vision of the EHR is that discrete data would be entered by providers into an EHR via:

    a. Codes

    b. COLD

    c. Digital dictation

    d. Templates

304. The key for linking data about an individual who is seen in a variety of care settings is:

    a. Facility medical record number

    b. Facility identification number

    c. Identity matching algorithm

    d. Patient birth date

305. Which statement is true concerning CDR and EHR?

    a. CDR supports management of data for an EHR.

    b. CDR and an EHR are the same.

    c. CDR is an early stage of EHR.

    d. CDR captures documents; EHR captures data.

306. The primary user of computerized provider order entry is:

    a. Nurse

    b. Patient

    c. Pharmacist

    d. Physician

307. One of the advantages of an EDMS is that it can:

    a. Help manage work tasks

    b. Decrease the time records should be retained

    c. Improve communications with physicians

    d. Eliminate all the problems encountered with the paper record

308. Which of the following computer architectures uses a single large computer to process data received from terminals into which data are entered?

    a. Client/server

    b. Local area network

    c. Mainframe

    d. Web services architecture

309. A transition technology used by many hospitals to increase access to medical record content is:

    a. Electronic health record

    b. Electronic document management system

    c. Electronic signature authentication

    d. Electronic data interchange

310. When a hospital develops its EHR system by selecting one vendor to provide financial and administrative applications and another vendor to supply the clinical applications, this is commonly referred to as a _____ strategy.

    a. Best-of-fit

    b. Best-of-breed

    c. Dual core

    d. Single source

311. Which of the following is *not* true about document imaging?

    a. Allows random access for retrieval of documents

    b. Can be viewed by more than one person at a time

    c. Can be viewed from locations remote from the HIM department

    d. Uses microfilm to store images

312. What type of information system would be used for processing patient admissions, employee time cards, and purchase orders?

    a. Decision support system

    b. Executive information system

    c. Management information system

    d. Transaction processing system

313. The first phase of the SDLC is the _____ phase.

    a. System design

    b. System testing

    c. Maintenance

    d. Planning

314. What basic components make up every electronic network communications system?

    a. Clients, peers, and servers

    b. Networks, browsers, and connections

    c. Transmitters, receivers, media, and data

    d. Hardware, software, data, and intranets

315. The concept of systems integration refers to the healthcare organization's ability to:

    a. Combine information from any system within the organization

    b. Use information from one system at a time

    c. Combine information from systems outside the organization

    d. Use information strictly for administrative purposes

316. The RFP generally includes a detailed description of the system's requirements and provides guidelines for vendors to follow in:

    a. Negotiating the price

    b. Demonstrating the product

    c. Bidding for the contract

    d. Setting up on-site demonstrations

317. The most common approaches to converting from an old information system to a new one are the parallel approach, the phased approach, and the _____ approach.

    a. Train-the-trainer

    b. Direct cutover

    c. Backup

    d. Upgrade

318. In which phase of the systems development life cycle is the primary focus on identifying and assigning priorities to the various upgrades and changes that might be made in an organization's information systems?

    a. Design

    b. Implementation

    c. Maintenance

    d. Planning

319. In which phase of the systems development life cycle are trial runs of the new system conducted, backup and disaster recover procedures developed, and training of end users performed?

    a. Design

    b. Implementation

    c. Maintenance and evaluation

    d. Planning and analysis

320. Which of the following is considered a consumer-centric informatics application?

    a. DSS

    b. EHR

    c. MIS

    d. PHR

321. Which of the following best describes the function of kiosks?

    a. A computer station that physicians can use to order medications

    b. A computer station that unlocks workstations

    c. A computer station that facilitates integrated communications within the healthcare organization

    d. A computer station that promotes the healthcare organization's services

322. A medication being ordered is contraindicated due to a patient allergy. The physician is notified. This is an example of a(n):

    a. Reminder

    b. Order entry/results reporting

    c. Alert

    d. Administrative decision support

323. Which of the following systems would the HIM department director use to receive daily reports on the number of new admissions to, and discharges from, the hospital?

    a. Transaction processing system

    b. Knowledge management system

    c. Management information system

    d. Decision support system

324. Which of the following is a snapshot in time and consolidates data from multiple sources to enhance decision making?

    a. CDW

    b. DSS

    c. KMS

    d. MIS

325. Which of the following uses artificial intelligence techniques to capture the knowledge of human experts and to translate and store it in a knowledge base?

    a. Database

    b. Data warehouse

    c. Expert system

    d. Management information system

326. Which of the following stores data in predefined tables consisting of rows and columns?

    a. Spreadsheet

    b. Relational database

    c. Hierarchical database

    d. Network database

327. Which of the following uniquely identifies each record in a database table?

    a. Data definition

    b. Data element

    c. Foreign key

    d. Primary key

328. What is the purpose of computer databases?

    a. Help computers communicate among themselves

    b. Connect computers together in a relatively small area

    c. Store and retrieve data

    d. Make the Internet accessible

329. Which of the following is a technique for graphically depicting the structure of a computer database?

    a. Data model

    b. Data flow diagram

    c. Foreign key

    d. Primary key

330. An organization identifies key people in various functional areas to be trained first, and then asks them to subsequently train other users in this same functional area. What is this approach to user training called?

    a. Action trainer

    b. Direct cutover approach

    c. Parallel training approach

    d. Train-the-trainer

331. Which of the following connects computers together in a way that allows for the sharing of information and resources?

    a. Network

    b. Client

    c. Transaction system

    d. Telephony

332. Which of the following is considered a two-factor authentication system?

    a. User ID with a password

    b. User ID with voice scan

    c. Password and swipe card

    d. Password and PIN

333. Which of the following technologies would reduce the risk that information is not accessible during a server crash?

    a. RAID

    b. Storage area network

    c. Server redundancy

    d. Tape or disk back-up

334. A system that enables processing of diagnostic studies results into tables, graphs, or other structures is:

    a. Results retrieval and management technology

    b. Data capture technology

    c. Clinical decision support

    d. Electronic document/content management

335. Community Hospital's hardware has been placed on back-order; the network team is having trouble getting the network to function properly. This is an example of:

    a. System build

    b. Issues management

    c. Integration testing

    d. Technical infrastructure

336. Audit logs and alert pop-ups are examples of:

    a. Metadata

    b. Encryption

    c. Admissibility

    d. Data integrity

337. Which of the following is a family of standards that aid the exchange of data among hospital systems and physician practices?

    a. CTI

    b. LAN

    c. HL7

    d. WAN

338. The following descriptors about the data element PATIENT_LAST_NAME are included in a data dictionary: definition: legal surname of the patient; field type: numeric; field length: 50; required field: yes; default value: none; input mask: none. Which of the following is true about the definition of this data element?

    a. The field type should be changed to Character.

    b. The input mask should be changed from None to Required.

    c. The field length should be shortened.

    d. A default value should be Required.

339. Systems testing of a new information system should be conducted using:

    a. Data supplied by the vendor

    b. Test data

    c. Actual patient data

    d. Data from the training database

340. Which of the following are used to associate relationships between entities (tables) in a relational database?

    a. Primary keys

    b. Unique identifiers

    c. Data attributes

    d. Foreign keys

341. Which of the following security controls are built into a computer software program?

    a. Physical controls

    b. Administration controls

    c. Application controls

    d. Media controls

342. Community Hospital is identifying strategies to minimize the security risks associated with employees leaving their workstations unattended. Which of the following solutions will minimize the security risk of unattended workstations?

    a. Use biometrics for access to the system.

    b. Implement firewall and virus protection.

    c. Implement session terminations.

    d. Install encryption and similar devices.

Domain V *Quality* Start: 10:30 am   End: 11:09

343. An HIM department is researching various options for scanning the hospital's health records. The department director would like to achieve efficiencies through scanning such as performing coding and cancer registry functions remotely. Given these considerations, which of the following would be the best scanning process?

    a. Scanning all documents at the time of patient discharge

    b. Scanning all documents after physicians have completed any record deficiencies

    c. Begin remote work only after all deficiencies have been corrected in the paper record

    d. Using scanners with the maximum amount of output

344. In conducting a qualitative analysis to ensure that documentation in the health record supports the diagnosis of the patient, what documentation would a coder look for to substantiate the diagnosis of aspiration pneumonia?

    a. Diffuse parenchymal lung disease on x-ray

    b. Patient has history of inhaled food, liquid, or oil

    c. Positive culture for *Pneumocystis carinii*

    d. Positive culture for *Streptococcus* pneumonia

345. Which of the following is an organization's planned response to protect its information in the case of a natural disaster?

    a. Administrative controls

    b. Audit trail

    c. Business continuity plan

    d. Physical controls

346. Which of the following is *not* a responsibility of a healthcare organization's quality management department?

    a. Helping departments to identify potential clinical quality problems

    b. Participating in regular departmental meetings across the organization

    c. Conducting medical peer review to identify patterns of care

    d. Determining the method for studying potential problems

347. Which of the following has the ultimate responsibility for ensuring quality in a healthcare facility?

    a. Board of Directors

    b. Quality management department

    c. Medical staff

    d. Utilization management department

348. The process that involves ongoing surveillance and prevention of infections so as to ensure the quality and safety of healthcare for patients and employees is known as:

    a. Utilization management

    b. Infection control

    c. Risk management

    d. Case management

349. Every healthcare organization's risk management plan should include the following components *except*:

    a. Loss prevention and reduction

    b. Safety and security management

    c. Peer review

    d. Claims management

350. Hospital A discharges 10,000 patients per year. Hospital B is located in the same town and discharges 5,000 patients per year. At Hospital B's medical staff committee meeting, a physician reports that he is concerned about the quality of care at Hospital B because the hospital has double the number of deaths per year than Hospital A. The HIM director is attending the meeting in a staff position. Which of the following actions should the director take?

    a. Make no comment since this is a medical staff meeting.

    b. Agree with the physician that the data suggest a quality issue.

    c. Suggest that the data be adjusted for possible differences in type and volume of patients treated.

    d. Suggest that an audit be done immediately to determine the cause of deaths within the hospital.

351. Which of the following provide process measure metrics in a precise format?

    a. Dashboard

    b. Scoreboard

    c. Structured indicator

    d. Outcome indicator

352. Total quality management and continuous quality improvement are well-known:

    a. Performance improvement models

    b. Quality indicators

    c. Change management techniques

    d. Management philosophies

353. Donabedian proposed three types of quality indicators: structure indicators, process indicators, and:

    a. Performance indicators

    b. Management indicators

    c. Outcome indicators

    d. Output indicators

354. Many organizations and quality experts define quality as meeting or exceeding:

    a. Patient quotas

    b. System outputs

    c. Customer expectations

    d. Data collection

355. Managing the adoption and implementation of new processes is called:

    a. Management by design

    b. Change management

    c. Process flow implementation

    d. Visioning

356. How do health plans incentivize providers to use EHRs?

    a. Denying paper claims

    b. Requiring external reporting

    c. Paying for performance programs

    d. Requiring use of clinical guidelines

357. A key feature of performance improvement is:

    a. Replacing unstructured decision making

    b. Developing managers to control processes

    c. An endless loop of feedback

    d. A continuous cycle of improvement

358. Brainstorming, affinity grouping, and nominal group techniques are tools and techniques used during performance improvement initiatives to facilitate _____ among employees.

    a. Communication

    b. Knowledge

    c. Quality improvement

    d. Cooperation

359. Periodic performance reviews:

    a. Encourage good performance

    b. Take the place of annual reviews

    c. Are the only opportunity to discuss performance

    d. Are only important when there are problems

360. Which of the following is a data collection tool that records current processes?

    a. Flow chart

    b. Force-field analysis

    c. Pareto chart

    d. Scatter diagram

361. According to the Pareto Principle:

    a. 20% of the sources of a problem are responsible for 80% of its actual effects

    b. 80% of the sources of a problem are responsible for 80% of its effects

    c. 20% of the sources of a problem are responsible for 20% of its effects

    d. 80% of the sources of a problem are responsible for 100% of its effects

362. Change management is the process of planning for change. It concentrates on:

    a. Addressing employee resistance to changes in processes, procedures, and policies

    b. Scheduling planned changes in processes, procedures, and policies

    c. Implementing the technology required to execute planned changes

    d. Managing the cost of implementing planned changes

363. Which of the following statements does *not* represent a fundamental principle of performance improvement?

    a. The structure of a system determines its performance.

    b. Systems are static and do not demonstrate variation.

    c. Improvements rely on the collection and analysis of data.

    d. Performance improvement requires the commitment and support of top administration.

364. Which of the following should be the first step in any quality improvement decision-making process?

    a. Analyzing the problem

    b. Identifying the problem

    c. Developing an alternative solution

    d. Deciding on the best solution

365. Community Hospital has compared its 2005 and 2011 admission type patient profile data. From a performance improvement standpoint, which admission types should the hospital examine for possible changes in capacity handling?

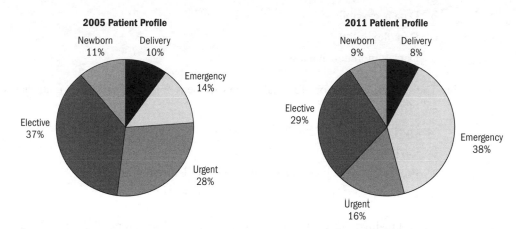

2005 Patient Profile

Newborn 11%
Delivery 10%
Emergency 14%
Elective 37%
Urgent 28%

2011 Patient Profile

Newborn 9%
Delivery 8%
Elective 29%
Emergency 38%
Urgent 16%

   a. Elective

   b. Emergency

   c. Newborn

   d. Urgent

366. As part of the clinic's performance improvement program, an HIM director wants to implement benchmarking for the transcription division at a large physician clinic. The clinic has 21 transcriptionists who average about 140 lines per hour. The transcription unit supports 80 physicians at a cost of 15 cents per line. What should be the first step that the supervisor takes to establish benchmarks for the transcription division?

   a. Clearly define what is to be studied and accomplished by instituting benchmarks.

   b. Hold a meeting with the transcriptionists to announce the benchmark program.

   c. Obtain benchmarks from other institutions.

   d. Hire a consultant to assist with the process.

367. A record that fails quantitative analysis is missing the quality criterion of:

   a. Legibility

   b. Reliability

   c. Completeness

   d. Clarity

368. A report that lists the ICD-9-CM codes associated with each physician in a healthcare facility can be used to assess the quality of the physician's services before he or she is:

   a. Scheduled for a coding audit

   b. Subjected to corrective action

   c. Recommended for staff reappointment

   d. Involved in an in-house training program

369. When all required data elements are included in the health record, the quality characteristic for _____ is met.

   a. Data security

   b. Data accessibility

   c. Data flexibility

   d. Data comprehensiveness

370. The sixth scope of work for quality improvement organizations (QIOs) introduced which of the following?

   a. Hospital Payment Monitoring Program

   b. Payment Error Prevention Program

   c. Program for Evaluation Payment Patterns Electronic Report

   d. Compliance Program Guidance for Hospitals

371. The following table compares Community Hospital's pneumonia length of stay (observed LOS) to the pneumonia LOS of similar hospitals (expected LOS). Given this data, where might Community Hospital want to focus attention on its pneumonia LOS?

LOS Summary for Pneumonia by Clinical Specialty				
Clinical Specialty	Cases	Observed LOS	Expected LOS	Savings Opportunity
Cardiology	1	6	6.36	0
Family Practice	17	8.47	6.26	38
Internal Medicine	34	3.82	4.89	−36
Endocrinology	1	3	3.93	−1
Pediatrics	7	3.43	3.55	−1

   a. Cardiology

   b. Endocrinology

   c. Family practice

   d. Internal medicine

372. After an outpatient review, individual audit results by coder should become part of the:

   a. Individual employee's performance evaluation

   b. Patient's health record

   c. Coding compliance review summary

   d. Mission of the coding team

373. The following data has been collected about the HIM department's coding productivity as part of the organization's total quality improvement program. Which of the following is the best assessment of this data?

Coder	Work Output (All Records Coded)	Total Hours Worked	Average Work Output per Hour	Completed Work Percentage	Completed Work Output (Records Coded Accurately)	Completed Work per Hour Worked
A	500	140 (full time)	3.57	91%	455	3.25
B	475	140 (full time)	3.39	96%	456	3.26
C	300	80 (part time)	3.75	85%	240	3.00
D	350	80 (part time)	4.69	70%	245	3.06
Department Average			3.69			3.17

> **Work Output:** Number of work units as recorded by the employee or the process
> **Total Hours Worked:** Number of hours worked by the employee to produce work, which does not include time on meals, breaks, and meetings
> **Average Work Output per Hour:** Work output divided by total hours worked
> **Completed Work Percentage:** Percentage of records coded accurately
> **Completed Work Output:** Work output multiplied by completed work percentage
> **Completed Work per Hour Worked:** Completed work output divided by total hours worked

a. Part-time coders are more productive than full-time coders.

b. Full-time coders are more productive than part-time coders.

c. All coders produce more than the departmental average.

d. Part-time coders exceed the departmental average.

374. The primary goal of the Hospital Standardization Program established in 1918 by the American College of Surgeons was to:

a. Establish minimum quality standards for hospitals.

b. Train physicians and nurses for American hospitals.

c. Standardize the educational curricula of American medical schools.

d. Force substandard hospitals to close.

375. A quantitative tool that provides an indication of an organization's performance in relation to a specified process or outcome is a(n):

    a. Performance measure

    b. Improvement opportunity

    c. Team-based process

    d. Data measure

376. A standard of performance or best practice for a particular process or outcome is called a(n):

    a. Performance measure

    b. Benchmark

    c. Improvement opportunity

    d. Data measure

377. This type of performance measure focuses on a process that leads to a certain outcome, meaning that a scientific or experiential basis exists for believing that the process, when executed well, will increase the probability of achieving a desired outcome.

    a. Outcome measure

    b. Data measure

    c. Process measure

    d. System measure

378. Which of the following is *not* a step in quality improvement decision-making?

    a. Determination of the quickest solution

    b. Definition of the problem

    c. Development of alternative solutions

    d. Implementation and follow-up

379. The principal process by which organizations optimize the continuum of care for their patients is:

    a. Utilization management

    b. Services management

    c. Case management

    d. Resource management

380. When the patient's physician contacts a healthcare organization to schedule an episode of care service, the healthcare organization begins which step in the case management process?

    a. Preadmission care planning

    b. Care planning at the time of admission

    c. Review the progress of care

    d. Discharge planning

381. The National Patient Safety Goals (NPSGs) have effectively mandated all healthcare organizations to examine care processes that have a potential for error that can cause injury to patients. Which of the following processes are included in the NPSGs?

    a. Identify patients correctly, prevent infection, and file claims for reimbursement

    b. Check patient medicines, prevent infection, and identify patients correctly

    c. File claims for reimbursement, check patient medicines, and improve staff communication

    d. Improve staff communication, process claims timely, and prevent infection

382. The interrelated activities in healthcare organizations, which promote effective and safe patient outcomes across services and disciplines within an integrated environment, are included in what area of performance measurement?

    a. Outcomes

    b. Processes

    c. Systems

    d. Benchmarks

383. A performance measure that enables healthcare organizations to monitor a process to determine whether it is meeting process requirements is called:

    a. Indicator

    b. Data measure

    c. Indication

    d. System measure

384. This status is conferred by a national professional organization that is dedicated to a specific area of healthcare practice.

    a. Credential

    b. Certificate

    c. License

    d. Degree

385. The primary objective of quality in healthcare for both patient and provider is to:

    a. Keep costs under control

    b. Reduce death rates

    c. Reduce the incidence of infectious diseases

    d. Arrive at the desired outcomes

386. Who is responsible for ensuring the quality of health record documentation?

    a. Board of directors

    b. Administrator

    c. Provider

    d. Health information management professional

387. All of the following services are typically reviewed for medical necessity and utilization *except*:

   a. Rehabilitative therapies

   b. Inpatient admissions

   c. Well-baby check

   d. Mental health and chemical dependency care

388. A Joint Commission–accredited organization must review its formulary annually to ensure a medication's continued:

   a. Safety and dose

   b. Efficiency and efficacy

   c. Efficacy and safety

   d. Dose and efficiency

389. Environmental assessments are performed as part of which of the following processes?

   a. Strategic planning

   b. Operational planning

   c. Quality improvement planning

   d. Budget planning

390. Which of the following actions is *not* included about a physician in the National Practitioner Data Bank?

   a. Malpractice lawsuits

   b. Disciplinary actions

   c. Credentialing information from other facilities

   d. Personal bankruptcy

391. The Joint Commission's quality improvement activities for health record documentation include all *but* which of the following core performance measures for hospitals:

   a. Acute myocardial infarction

   b. Hypertension

   c. Pregnancy and related conditions

   d. Seizure disorder

392. This data set was developed by the National Committee for Quality Assurance to aid consumers with health-related issues with information to compare performance of clinical measures for health plans:

   a. HEDIS

   b. UHDDS

   c. UACDS

   d. ORYX

393. In this case management step, the case manager confirms that the patient meets criteria for the care setting and that the services can be provided at the facility.

    a. Preadmission care planning

    b. Care planning at the time of admission

    c. Review the progress of care

    d. Discharge planning

394. The final results of care, treatment, and services in terms of the patient's expectations, needs, and quality of life, which may be positive and appropriate or negative and diminishing, are included in what area of performance measurement?

    a. Outcomes

    b. Processes

    c. Systems

    d. Benchmarks

395. An established set of clinical decisions and actions taken by clinicians and other representatives of healthcare organizations in accordance with state and federal laws, regulations, and guidelines is called:

    a. Standards of care

    b. Clinical practice standards

    c. Clinical pathways

    d. Standard guidelines

396. An HIM director reviews the departmental scanning productivity reports for the past three months and sees that productivity is below that of the national average. Which of the following actions should the director take?

    a. Reduce the salary of the non-productive workers.

    b. Investigate whether there are factors contributing to the low productivity that are not reflected in the national benchmarks.

    c. Meet with departmental supervisors to discuss the issue.

    d. Assess whether or not the current economy is affecting productivity.

397. Through the establishment of the National Practitioner Data Bank, the federal government became involved in malpractice issues and what other type of issue?

    a. Employment of physicians

    b. Quality of care

    c. Licensure of physicians

    d. Pay for performance

398. All of the following are Joint Commission core measure criteria sets *except*:

    a. Heart failure

    b. Acute myocardial infarction

    c. Pneumonia

    d. Diabetes mellitus

399. During training, the employee should be:

   a. Allowed to work without supervision

   b. Expected to make no mistakes

   c. Evaluated to make sure work is error free

   d. Evaluated for productivity

400. Community Hospital performed a cost-savings analysis between its current paper-based, on-site coding processes and an e-WebCoding telecommuting model. Given the graph here, what does the cost analysis show?

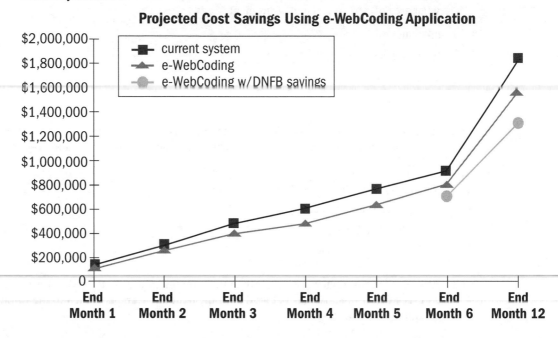

Projected Cost Savings Using e-WebCoding Application

   a. Current system saves more than the e-WebCoding system

   b. Current system reduces DNFB significantly

   c. Cost comparison reflects a net reduction in overall expenses on a monthly basis for the e-WebCoding system

   d. e-WebCoding consistently costs the hospital more than the current system

401. A coding supervisor who makes up the weekly work schedule would engage in what type of planning?

   a. Long-range

   b. Operational

   c. Tactical

   d. Strategic

402. Performance standards are used to:

a. Communicate performance expectations

b. Assign daily work

c. Describe the elements of a job

d. Prepare a job advertisement

403. A supervisor wants to determine whether the release of information staff are working at optimal output. Which of the following would be most useful to determine this?

a. Review work attendance records to see who is absent from work the most.

b. Walk through the work area at random times of the day to make sure that employees are at their desks and working.

c. Set productivity standards for the area and review results on a regular basis.

d. Determine the backlog of work not performed each day.

404. I reviewed the patient's record of Mr. Brown and found there was no H&P on the record at seven hours past this patient's admission time. This would be an example of:

a. Quantitative analysis

b. Qualitative analysis

c. Data mining

d. Data warehousing

405. I reviewed the health record of Sally Williams and found the physician stated on her post-op note, "examined after surgery." This would be an example of:

a. Quantitative analysis

b. Qualitative analysis

c. Data mining

d. Data warehousing

Domain VI *Legal* Start 12:39 pm End: 1:06 pm

406. Attorneys for healthcare organizations use the health record to:

a. Support claims for medical malpractice

b. Protect the legal interests of the facility and its healthcare providers

c. Plan and market services

d. Locate missing persons

407. Under HIPAA, which of the following is *not* named as a covered entity?

a. Outsourced transcription company

b. Health plan

c. Healthcare clearinghouse

d. Healthcare provider

408. The HIPAA Privacy Rule:

a. Protects only medical information that is not already specifically protected by state law

b. Supersedes all state laws that conflict with it

c. Is federal common law

d. Sets a minimum (floor) of privacy requirements

409. A competent individual has the following rights in regard to his or her healthcare:

a. Right to consent to treatment and the right to destroy their original health record

b. Right to destroy their original health record and the right to refuse treatment

c. Right to access his or her own PHI and the right to take the original record with them

d. Right to consent to treatment and the right to access his or her own PHI

410. Which of the following is *not* an element that makes information "PHI" under the HIPAA Privacy Rule?

a. Identifies an individual

b. In the custody of or transmitted by a CE or its BA

c. Contained within a personnel file

d. Relates to one's health condition

411. Which of the following is *not* an identifier under the Privacy Rule?

a. Visa account 2773 985 0468

b. Vehicle license plate BZ LITYR

c. Age 75

c. Street address 265 Cherry Valley Road

412. Central City Clinic has requested that Ghent Hospital send its hospital records from Susan Hall's most recent admission to the clinic for her follow-up appointment. Which of the following statements is true?

a. The Privacy Rule requires that Susan Hall complete a written authorization.

b. The hospital may send only discharge summary, history and physical, and operative report.

c. The Privacy Rule's minimum necessary requirement does not apply.

d. This "public interest and benefit" disclosure does not require the patient's authorization.

413. Susan is completing her required high school community service hours by serving as a volunteer at the local hospital. Relative to the hospital, she is a(n):

a. Business associate

b. Employee

c. Workforce member

d. Covered entity

414. Lane Hospital has a contract with Ready-Clean, a local company, to come into the hospital to pick up all of the facility's linens for off-site laundering. Ready-Clean is:

    a. A business associate because Lane Hospital has a contract with it

    b. Not a business associate because it is a local company

    c. A business associate because its employees may see PHI

    d. Not a business associate because it does not use or disclose individually identifiable health information

415. Jeremy Lykins was required to undergo a physical exam prior to becoming employed by San Fernando Hospital. Jeremy's medical information is:

    a. Protected by the Privacy Rule because it is individually identifiable

    b. Not protected by the Privacy Rule because it is part of a personnel record

    c. Protected by the Privacy Rule because it contains his physical exam results

    d. Protected by the Privacy Rule because it is in the custody of a covered entity

416. The HIPAA Security Awareness and Training administrative safeguard requires all of the following addressable implementation programs for an entity's workforce *except*:

    a. Disaster recovery plan

    b. Log-in monitoring

    c. Password management

    d. Security reminders

417. Burning, shredding, pulping, and pulverizing are *all* acceptable methods in which process?

    a. Deidentification of electronic documents

    b. Destruction of paper-based health records

    c. Deidentification of records stored on mircofilm

    d. Destruction of computer-based health records

418. Which of the following data sets would be most useful in developing a grid for identification of components of the legal health record in a hybrid record environment?

    a. Document name, media type, source system, electronic storage start date, stop printing start date

    b. Document name, media type

    c. Document name, medical record number, source system

    d. Document name, source system

419. The _____ provide the objective and scope for the HIPAA Security Rule as a whole.

    a. Administrative provisions

    b. General rules

    c. Physical safeguards

    d. Technical safeguards

420. Which of the following must covered entities do to comply with HIPAA security provisions?

    a. Appoint an individual who has the title of chief security officer who is responsible for security management

    b. Conduct employee security training sessions every six months for all employees

    c. Establish a contingency plan

    d. Conduct technical and nontechnical evaluations every six years

421. For HIPAA implementation specifications that are addressable, which of the following statements is true?

    a. The implementation specification must be implemented by the covered entity.

    b. The covered entity may choose not to implement the specification if implementation is too costly.

    c. The covered entity must conduct a risk assessment to determine whether the specification is appropriate to its environment.

    d. If the covered entity is a small hospital, the specification does not have to be implemented.

422. The medical record of Kathy Smith, the plaintiff, has been subpoenaed for a deposition. The plaintiff's attorney wishes to use the records as evidence to prove his client's case. In this situation, although the record constitutes hearsay, it may be used as evidence based on the:

    a. Admissibility exception

    b. Discovery exception

    c. Direct evidence exception

    d. Business records exception

423. From an evidentiary standpoint, incident reports:

    a. Should not be placed in a patient's health record

    b. May be referenced in the patient's health record

    c. Are universally non-admissible during trial proceedings

    d. Are universally non-discoverable during litigation

424. A hospital employee destroyed a health record so that its contents—which would be damaging to the employee—could not be used at trial. In legal terms, the employee's action constitutes:

    a. Mutilation

    b. Destruction

    c. Spoliation

    d. Spoilage

425. Authentication of a record refers to:

    a. Establishment of its baseline trustworthiness

    b. The type of electronic operating system on which it was created

    c. The identity of the individual who notarized it

    d. Its relevance

426. When served with a court order directing the release of health records, an individual:

   a. May ignore it

   b. Must comply with it

   c. Must request patient authorization before disclosing the records

   d. May determine whether or not to comply with it

427. The following step should *not* be included in a health information department's procedure for preparing health records in response to a subpoena:

   a. Number the pages

   b. Remove pages containing detrimental information

   c. Photocopy the record

   d. Ensure the patient's name is present on every page

428. Written or spoken permission to proceed with care is classified as:

   a. An advanced directive

   b. Formal consent

   c. Expressed consent

   d. Implied consent

429. To be in compliance with HIPAA regulations, a hospital would make its membership in a RHIO known to its patients through which of the following?

   a. Press release

   b. Notice of Privacy Practices

   c. Consent form

   d. Website notice

430. Law enacted by a legislative body is a(n):

   a. Administrative law

   b. Statute

   c. Regulation

   d. Rule

431. What is the legal term used to describe the physical and electronic protection of health information?

   a. Access

   b. Confidentiality

   c. Privacy

   d. Security

432. The "custodian of health records" refers to the individual within an organization who is responsible for the following action(s), *except:*

    a. Authorized to certify records

    b. Supervises inspection and copying of record

    c. Testifies to the authenticity of records

    d. Testifies regarding the care of the patient

433. Who owns the health record?

    a. Patient

    b. Provider who generated the information

    c. Insurance company who paid for the care recorded in the record

    d. No one

434. The process of releasing health record documentation originally created by a different provider is called:

    a. Privileged communication

    b. Subpoena

    c. Jurisdiction

    d. Redisclosure

435. Which of the following is *not* true of notices of privacy practices?

    a. Must be made available at the site where the individual is treated.

    b. Must be posted in a prominent place.

    c. Must contain content that may not be changed.

    d. Must be prominently posted on the covered entity's website when the entity has one.

436. Which document directs an individual to bring originals or copies of records to court?

    a. Summons

    b. Subpoena

    c. Subpoena *duces tecum*

    d. Deposition

437. To comply with HIPAA, under usual circumstances, a covered entity must act on a patient's request to review or copy his or her health information within _____ days.

    a. 10

    b. 20

    c. 30

    d. 60

438. The HIPAA Privacy Rule requires that covered entities must limit use, access, and disclosure of PHI to only the amount needed to accomplish the intended purpose. What concept is this an example of?

    a. Minimum necessary

    b. Notice of privacy practices

    c. Authorization

    d. Consent

439. Which of the following statements is *false*?

    a. A notice of privacy practices must be written in plain language.

    b. A notice of privacy practices must have a statement that other uses and disclosures will be made only with the individual's written authorization and that the individual may revoke such authorization.

    c. An authorization does not have to be obtained for uses and disclosures for treatment, payment, and operations.

    d. A notice of privacy practices must give an example of a use or disclosure for healthcare operations.

440. The legal term used to describe when a patient has the right to maintain control over certain personal information is referred to as:

    a. Access

    b. Confidentiality

    c. Privacy

    d. Security

441. What is the legal term used to define the protection of health information in a patient-provider relationship?

    a. Access

    b. Confidentiality

    c. Privacy

    d. Security

442. Which of the following statements is *not* true about a business associate agreement?

    a. It prohibits the business associate from using or disclosing PHI for any purpose other than that described in the contract with the covered entity.

    b. It allows the business associate to maintain PHI indefinitely.

    c. It prohibits the business associate from using or disclosing PHI in any way that would violate the HIPAA Privacy Rule.

    d. It requires the business associate to make available all of its books and records relating to PHI use and disclosure to the Department of Health and Human Services or its agents.

443. Under HIPAA regulations, how many days does a covered entity have to respond to an individual's request for access to his or her PHI when the PHI is stored off-site?

    a. 10 days beyond the original requirement

    b. 30 days

    c. 60 days

    d. 90 days

444. The security officer is responsible for:

    a. Protecting PHI

    b. Advising administration on information security

    c. Monitoring patient rights

    d. Releasing PHI

445. Which of the following is an example of a business associate?

    a. Contract coder

    b. Environmental services

    c. Security officer

    d. Employee with access to e-PHI

446. What type of health record policy dictates how long individual health records must remain available for authorized use?

    a. Disclosure policies

    b. Legal policies

    c. Retention policies

    d. Redisclosure policies

447. If a patient wants to amend his or her health record, the covered entity may require the individual to:

    a. Make an amendment request in writing and provide a rationale for the amendment.

    b. Ask the attending physician for his or her permission to amend their record.

    c. Require the patient to wait 30 days before their request will be considered and processed.

    d. Provide a court order requesting the amendment.

448. Which of the following statements about the directory of patients maintained by a covered entity is true?

    a. Individuals must be given an opportunity to restrict or deny permission to place information about them in the directory.

    b. Individuals must provide a written authorization before information about them can be placed in the directory.

    c. The directory may contain only identifying information such as the patient's name and birth date.

    d. The directory may contain private information as long as it is kept confidential.

449. According to HIPAA, what does the abbreviation PHI stand for?

    a. Personal health information

    b. Protected health information

    c. Primary health information

    d. Past health information

450. Which of the following is *not* true about the Notice of Privacy Practices?

    a. Must include at least two examples of how information is used for both treatment and operations

    b. Must include a description of the right to request restrictions on certain uses and disclosures

    c. Must explain the patient's right to inspect and copy PHI

    d. Must include a description of the patient's right to amend PHI

451. The legal health record (LHR) is a(n):

    a. Defined subset of all patient-specific data created or accumulated by a healthcare provider that may be released to third parties in response to a legally permissible request for patient information

    b. Entire set of information created or accumulated by a healthcare provider that may be released to third parties in response to a legally permissible request for patient information

    c. Set of patient-specific data created or accumulated by a healthcare provider that is defined to be legal by the local, state, or federal authorities

    d. Set of patient-specific data that is defined to be legal by state or federal statute and that is legally permissible to provide in response to requests for patient information

452. When a patient revokes authorization for release of information *after* a healthcare facility has already released the information, the facility in this case:

    a. May be prosecuted for invasion of privacy

    b. Has become subject to civil action

    c. Has violated the security regulations of HIPAA

    d. Is protected by the Privacy Act

453. Which of the following has access to personally identifiable data without authorization or subpoena?

    a. Insurance company for life insurance eligibility

    b. The patient's attorney

    c. Public health department for disease reporting purposes

    d. Workers' compensation for disability claim settlement

454. Which of the following statements represents an example of nonmaleficence?

    a. HITs must ensure that patient-identifiable information is not released to unauthorized parties.

    b. HITs must apply rules fairly and consistently to every case.

    c. HITs must ensure that patient-identifiable information is released to the parties who need it to provide services to their patients.

    d. HITs must ensure that patients themselves, and not other parties, are authorizing access to the patients' individual health information.

455. An organization is served with a subpoena. An appropriate response to the reasonable anticipation of litigation would be to:

   a. Destroy all records associated with the anticipated litigation.

   b. Distribute copies of records associated with the anticipated litigation to all parties involved.

   c. Make a copy of the paper-based record associated with the anticipated litigation and give the original paper-based record to the organization's legal counsel to be secured in a locked file.

   d. Give all records associated with the anticipated litigation to the organization's legal counsel to be secured in a locked file.

456. Which organization issues and maintains ethical standards for the health information management profession?

   a. American Medical Association

   b. American Health Information Management Association

   c. American College of Surgeons

   d. American Hospital Association

457. The sister of a patient requests the HIM department to release copies of her brother's health record to her. She states that because the doctor documented her name as her brother's caregiver that HIPAA regulations apply and that she may receive copies of her brother's health record. In this case, how should the HIM department proceed?

   a. Provide the copies as requested since the sister was a caregiver.

   b. Provide only copies of the reports where the sister's name is mentioned.

   c. Refuse the request.

   d. Refer the individual to legal counsel.

458. Community Hospital is discussing restricting the access that physicians have to electronic clinical records. The medical record committee is divided on how to approach this issue. Some committee members maintain that all information should be available, whereas others maintain that HIPAA restricts access. The HIM director is part of the committee. Which of the following should the director advise the committee?

   a. HIPAA restricts the access of physicians to all information.

   b. The "minimum necessary" concept does not apply to disclosures made for treatment purposes; therefore physician access should not be restricted.

   c. The "minimum necessary" concept does not apply to disclosures made for treatment purposes, but the organization must define what physicians need as part of their treatment role.

   d. The "minimum necessary" concept applies only to attending physicians and therefore restriction of access must be implemented.

459. A physician takes the medical records of a group of HIV-positive patients out of the hospital to complete research tasks at home. The physician mistakenly leaves the records in a restaurant, where they are read by a newspaper reporter who publishes an article that identifies the patients. The physician can be sued for:

   a. Slander

   b. Willful infliction of mental distress

   c. Libel

   d. Invasion of privacy

460. Mrs. Bolton is an angry patient who resents her physicians "bossing her around." She refuses to take a portion of the medications the nurses bring to her pursuant to physician orders and is verbally abusive to the patient care assistants. Of the following options, the most appropriate way to document Mrs. Bolton's behavior in the patient medical record is:

a. Mean

b. Non-compliant and hostile toward staff

c. Belligerent and out of line

d. A pain in the neck

461. As the corporate director of HIM Services and enterprise privacy officer, you are asked to review a patient's health record in preparation for a legal proceeding for a malpractice case. The lawsuit was brought by the patient 72 days after the procedure. Health information contains a summary of two procedures that were dictated 95 days after the procedure. The physician in question has a longstanding history of being lackadaisical with record completion practices. Previous concerns regarding this physician's record maintenance practices had been reported to the facility's Credentialing Committee. Is this information admissible in court?

a. This information could be rejected since the physician dictated the procedure note after the malpractice suit was filed.

b. This information will be admissible in court because it is part of the patient's health record.

c. This information could be rejected because it is not relevant to the malpractice case.

d. This information will be rejected because the patient did not authorize its release.

462. While auditing health records for incomplete documentation, the HIM specialist identifies written progress notes by Dr. Doe that she cannot read. She reports this to the hospital's risk manager. What is the best method to determine the scope of the documentation problem by Dr. Doe?

a. An HIM professional should conduct a more detailed audit of Dr. Doe's patients' records.

b. Suspend Dr. Doe for his illegible documentation.

c. Report Dr. Doe to the medical director.

d. Contact the compliance hotline and revoke Dr. Doe's privileges.

Domain VII *Revenue Cycle*   Start: 12:10 pm   End: 12:37 pm.

463. A Medicare patient had two physician office visits, underwent hospital radiology examinations, clinical laboratory tests, and received take-home surgical dressings. Which of the following could be reimbursed under the outpatient prospective payment system?

a. Clinical laboratory tests

b. Physician office visits

c. Radiology examinations

d. Take-home surgical dressings

464. In conducting a qualitative review, the clinical documentation specialist sees that the nursing staff has documented the patient's skin integrity on admission to support the presence of a stage I pressure ulcer. However, the physician's documentation is unclear as to whether this condition was present on admission. How should the clinical documentation specialist proceed?

   a. Note the condition as present on admission.

   b. Query the physician to determine if the condition was present on admission.

   c. Note the condition as unknown on admission.

   d. Note the condition as not present on admission.

465. Given the following information, from which payer does the hospital proportionately receive the least amount of payment?

Payer	Charges	Payments	Adjustments	Charges	Payments	Adjustments
BC/BS	$450,000	$360,000	$90,000	23%	31%	12%
Commercial	$250,000	$200,000	$50,000	13%	17%	6%
Medicaid	$350,000	$75,000	$275,000	18%	6%	36%
Medicare	$750,000	$495,000	$255,000	39%	42%	33%
TRICARE	$150,000	$50,000	$100,000	7%	4%	13%
Total	$1,950,000	$1,180,000	$770,000	100%	100%	100%

   a. BC/BS

   b. Medicaid

   c. Medicare

   d. TRICARE

466. Which of the following is the definition of revenue cycle management?

   a. The regularly repeating set of events that produce revenue or income

   b. The method by which patients are grouped together based on a set of characteristics

   c. The systematic comparison of the products, services, and outcomes of one organization with those of a similar organization

   d. Coordination of all administrative and clinical functions that contribute to the capture, management, and collection of patient service revenue

467. Most facilities begin counting days in accounts receivable at which of the following times?

   a. The date the patient registers

   b. The date the patient is discharged

   c. The date the bill drops

   d. The date the bill is received by the payer

468. The amount of money owed a healthcare facility when claims are pending is called:

   a. Dollars in accounts receivable

   b. Bad debt

   c. The write-off account

   d. Delayed revenue

469. In a typical acute-care setting, the Explanation of Benefits, Medicare Summary Notice, and Remittance Advice documents (provided by the payer) are monitored in which revenue cycle area?

    a. Pre-claims submission

    b. Claims processing

    c. Accounts receivable

    d. Claims reconciliation/collections

470. Most chief financial officers view the HIM department's most essential role in the revenue cycle management to be:

    a. Assembly and abstraction of the record

    b. Coding of the record

    c. Medical transcription

    d. Release of information requested

471. When all third-party payments have been received and contractual allowances have been written off, the remaining balance is categorized as the patient responsibility. Best practice is to have the patient responsibility amount be less than what percentage of the total balance?

    a. 10

    b. 15

    c. 20

    d. 25

472. Which of the following types of hospitals are excluded from the Medicare inpatient prospective payment system?

    a. Children's

    b. Rural

    c. State supported

    d. Tertiary

473. When a provider agrees to accept of assignment from Medicare, the provider has agreed to:

    a. Reimbursement at 15% above the allowed charge

    b. Payment according to the MFS plus 10%

    c. Not bill patients for the balance

    d. Be referred to as a nonparticipating provider

474. In processing a Medicare payment for outpatient radiology exams, a hospital outpatient services department would receive payment under which of the following?

    a. DRGs

    b. HHRGS

    c. OASIS

    d. OPPS

475. Which of the following is *not* reimbursed according to the Medicare outpatient prospective payment system?

    a. CMHC partial hospitalization services

    b. Critical access hospitals

    c. Hospital outpatient departments

    d. Vaccines provided by CORFs

476. How often are the Medicare fee schedules updated?

    a. Annually

    b. Monthly

    c. Semiannually

    d. Weekly

477. Which of the following would a health record technician use to perform the billing function for a physician's office?

    a. Screen 837P or CMS 1500

    b. UB-04

    c. UB-92

    d. Screen 8371 or UB-04

478. When a provider accepts assignment, this means that the:

    a. Patient authorizes payment to be made directly to the provider

    b. Provider accepts as payment in full the allowed charge from the fee schedule

    c. Balance filling is allowed on patient accounts, but at a limited rate

    d. Participating provider receives a fee-for-service reimbursement

479. The coordination of benefits transaction (COB) is important so that:

    a. There is no duplication of benefits paid

    b. The hospital receives the full amount of billed services

    c. The provider receives the full amount of billed services

    d. The patient receives the correct bill

480. Community Hospital has launched a clinical documentation improvement (CDI) initiative. Currently, clinical documentation does not always adequately reflect the severity of illness of the patient or support optimal HIM coding accuracy. Given this situation, which of the following would be the best action to validate that the new program is achieving its goals?

    a. Hire clinical documentation specialists to review records prior to coding

    b. Ask coders to query physicians more often

    c. Provide physicians the opportunity to add addenda to their reports to clarify documentation issues

    d. Conduct a retrospective review of all query opportunities for the year

481. Which of the following is made up of claims data from Medicare claims submitted by acute-care hospitals and skilled nursing facilities?

    a. NPDB

    b. MEDPAR

    c. HIPDB

    d. UHDDS

482. The collection of information on healthcare fraud and abuse was mandated by HIPAA and resulted in the development of:

    a. National Practitioner Data Bank

    b. Healthcare Integrity and Protection Data Bank

    c. National Health Provider Inventory

    d. Nationwide False Claims Data Bank

483. What is the name of the federally funded program that pays the medical bills of the spouses and dependents of persons on active duty in the uniformed services?

    a. HHS-CMS

    b. TRICARE

    c. CHAMPVA

    d. Medigap

484. Mr. Jones is a 67-year-old patient who only has Medicare's Part A insurance. Given the information here, if Mr. Jones used 36 lifetime reserve days, how many does the patient have left to be used at a later date?

Date Admitted	Date Discharged
01/01	01/13
03/20	03/30
07/04	11/02
12/01	12/05

    a. 24 days

    b. 50 days

    c. 60 days

    d. 90 days

485. Under outpatient prospective payment system, Medicare decides how much a hospital or a community mental health center will be reimbursed for each service rendered. Depending on the service, the patient pays either a coinsurance amount (20%) or a fixed copayment amount, whichever is less. Mr. Smith, who has paid his deductible for the year, was charged $85 for a minor procedure performed in the hospital outpatient department. The fixed copayment amount for this type of procedure, adjusted for wages in the geographic area, is $15. What would Mr. Smith need to pay in this case?

    a. $15

    b. $17

    c. $68

    d. $85

486. The number of days Medicare will cover SNF inpatient care per benefit period is limited to which of the following?

    a. 21

    b. 60

    c. 30

    d. 100

487. Which of the following types of care is *not* covered by Medicare?

    a. Long-term nursing care

    b. Skilled nursing care

    c. Hospice care

    d. Home healthcare

488. Active armed services members and their qualified family members are covered by which of the following healthcare programs?

    a. Medicaid

    b. Medicare

    c. PACE

    d. TRICARE

489. What is the name of the program funded by the federal government to provide medical care to people on low incomes or with limited financial resources?

    a. CHAMPUS

    b. Medicare

    c. Medicaid

    d. Medigap

490. Some services are covered and paid by Medicare before Medicaid makes payments because Medicaid is considered which of the following?

    a. Qualified beneficiary

    b. Premium payer

    c. Payer of last resort

    d. Alternative payer

491. Which of the following groups of healthcare providers contracts with a self-insured employer to provide healthcare services?

    a. Preferred provider organization

    b. Health maintenance organization

    c. Point-of-service provider

    d. Independent Practice Association

492. Which of the following reimbursement methods pays providers according to charges that are calculated before healthcare services are rendered?

    a. Fee-for-service reimbursement method

    b. Prospective payment method

    c. Retrospective payment method

    d. Resource-based payment method

493. Which of the following apply to radiological and other procedures that include professional and technical components and are paid as a lump sum to be divided between physician and healthcare facility?

    a. Global payments

    b. Professional payment

    c. Bundled payment

    d. Fee-for-service

494. In a typical acute-care setting, which revenue cycle area uses an internal auditing system (scrubber) to ensure that error-free claims (clean claims) are submitted to third-party payers?

    a. Pre-claims submission

    b. Claims processing

    c. Accounts receivable

    d. Claims reconciliation/collections

495. Which entity is responsible for processing Part A claims and hospital-based Part B claims for institutional services on behalf of Medicare?

    a. Fiscal intermediary/MAC

    b. Medicare carrier

    c. Third-party payer

    d. Claim editor

496. Which of the following is a common registration error that will affect the revenue cycle?

    a. Transposed digits in the social security number, date of birth, or policy number

    b. Inaccurate laboratory results

    c. Discharge summary dictated more than 30 days post discharge

    d. Medication dosage error on prescription

497. In a typical acute-care setting, charge capture is located in which revenue cycle area?

   a. Pre-claims submission

   b. Claims processing

   c. Accounts receivable

   d. Claims reconciliation/collections

498. Which of the following establish eligibility standards for enrollment in Medicaid?

   a. Centers for Medicare and Medicaid Services

   b. Department of Health and Human Services

   c. Federal government

   d. Individual states

499. This program provides additional federal funds to states so that Medicaid eligibility can be expanded to include a greater number of children.

   a. Medigap

   b. PACE

   c. SCHIP

   d. TRICARE

500. The charge description master relieves the HIM department of _____ that does not require documentation analysis.

   a. Repetitive coding

   b. Manual coding

   c. Duplicate coding

   d. Procedure coding

501. After a claim has been filed with Medicare, a healthcare organization had late charges posted to a patient's outpatient account that changed the calculation of the APC. What is best practice for this organization to receive the correct reimbursement from Medicare?

   a. Nothing, because the claim has already been submitted

   b. Bill the patient for any remaining balance after payment from Medicare is received

   c. Submit an adjusted claim to Medicare

   d. Return the account to coding for review

502. Which term refers to the electronic transmission of information from a provider to a health plan to determine a patient's eligibility for services?

   a. Accounts payable

   b. Claims transaction

   c. Coordination of benefits transaction

   d. Accounts receivable

503. Which of the following agencies is responsible for providing healthcare services to American Indians and Alaska natives?

    a. CMS

    b. IHS

    c. NIH

    d. VA

504. Which of the following insurance covers healthcare costs and lost income associated with work-related injuries?

    a. CHAMPVA

    b. Medicare

    c. Medicaid

    d. Workers' compensation

505. A Medicare benefit period is defined as:

    a. Beginning the day the Medicare patient is admitted to the hospital and ending when the patient has been out of the hospital for 60 days in a row, including the day of discharge

    b. The period in which a Medicare or Medicaid patient is hospitalized

    c. The period that begins on January 1 of each year with an allowable inpatient hospitalization benefit of up to 90 days

    d. Between 1 and 90 days of a Medicare patient's hospitalization

506. City Hospital's RCM team has established the following benchmarks: (1) The value of discharged not final billed cases should not exceed two days of average daily revenue, and (2) AR days are not to exceed 60 days. The net average daily revenue is $1,000,000. What do the following data indicate about how City Hospital is meeting its benchmarks?

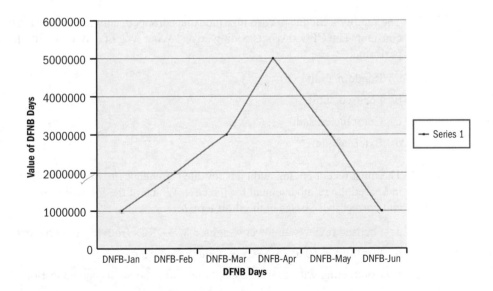

    a. DNFB cases met the benchmark 100% of the time.

    b. DNFB cases met the benchmark 75% of the time.

    c. DNFB cases met the benchmark 50% of the time.

    d. DNFB cases met the benchmark 25% of the time.

507. The patient's account balance is displaying a negative balance. What should the healthcare organization do to resolve this situation?

    a. Determine which payer overpaid and return the funds

    b. Do nothing because overpayment and underpayments balance out

    c. Wait for the payer to contact them about the overpayment

    d. Return the overpayment to payer who paid last on the claim

508. The unique number that identifies each service or supply in the CDM and links each item to a particular department is known as the:

    a. Revenue code

    b. General ledger key

    c. Charge code

    d. Item description

509. All of the following are required elements of a charge description master *except*:

    a. General ledger key

    b. Revenue code

    c. Charges

    d. Date of service

510. The codes used in a charge description master are:

    a. ICD-9-CM

    b. CPT-4

    c. HCPCS Levels I and II

    d. SNOMED CT

511. The facility's Medicare case-mix index has dropped, although other statistical measures appear constant. The CFO suspects coding errors. What type of coding quality review should be performed?

    a. Random audit

    b. Focused audit

    c. Compliance audit

    d. External audit

512. The most recent coding audit has revealed a tendency to miss secondary diagnoses that would have increased the reimbursement for the case. Which of the following strategies will help to identify and correct these cases in the short term?

    a. Focused reviews on lower weighted MS-DRGs from triples and pairs

    b. Facility top 10 to 15 APCs by volume and charges

    c. Contracting with a larger consulting firm to do audits and education

    d. Focused reviews on surgical complications

513. There should be four primary percentages that should be calculated and tracked to assess clinical documentation improvement (CDI) programs. These include all of the following *except*:

    a. Record review rate

    b. Query rate

    c. Query agreement rate

    d. Record agreement rate

514. CDI staff should revisit cases:

    a. Every day

    b. Weekly

    c. Every 48 hours

    d. Every 24 to 48 hours

515. The federal legislation that focused on healthcare fraud and abuse issues, especially as they relate to penalties, was the:

    a. Civil False Claims Act

    b. Health Insurance Portability and Accountability Act (HIPAA)

    c. Balanced Budget Act of 1997

    d. Gramm-Leach-Bliley Act

516. Which of the following services would be included in the 72-hour payment window and included in the inpatient MS-DRG payment to an acute-care hospital?

    a. Ambulance services

    b. Diagnostic laboratory testing

    c. Home health services

    d. Maintenance renal dialysis services

517. The phrase "bad debt" refers to accounts that include money owed by the patient and are:

    a. Overdue by 90 days and are in process of being referred to collections

    b. Paid in monthly installments under a payment agreement

    c. Determined by the facility to be uncollectible

    d. Waiting to be paid by the insurance company or third-party payer

518. The best practice for a system hold for all charges to be entered into the billing system and all coding to be completed is:

    a. 2 days post-discharge or visit

    b. 4 days post-discharge or visit

    c. 7 days post-discharge or visit

    d. 14 days post-discharge or visit

519. The "discharged, not final billed" report (also known as "discharged, no final bill" or "accounts not selected for billing") includes what types of accounts?

a. Accounts that have been discharged and have not been billed for a variety of reasons

b. Only discharged inpatient accounts awaiting generation of the bill

c. Only uncoded patient records

d. Accounts that are within the system hold days and not eligible to be billed

520. Patient Accounts has submitted a report to the revenue cycle team detailing $100,000 of outpatient accounts that are failing NCD edits. All attempts to clear the edits have failed. There are no ABNs on file for these accounts. Based only on this information, the revenue cycle team should:

a. Bill the patients for these accounts

b. Contact the patients to obtain an ABN

c. Write off the accounts to contractual allowances

d. Write off the failed charges to bad debt and bill Medicare for the clean charges

EXAM 1

Start: 7:00 pm   End: 8:17

Domain I *Data Analysis and Management*

1. A health record technician has been asked to review the discharge patient abstracting portion of a proposed new computer system. Which of the following data sets would the technician consult to ensure the system collects all the federally required data elements for discharged Medicare and Medicaid inpatients in an acute-care hospital?

   a. DEEDS
   b. CARF
   c. UACDS
   d. UHDDS

2. An outpatient clinic is reviewing the functionality of a computer system it is considering purchasing. Which of the following data sets should the clinic consult to ensure that all the federally recommended data elements for Medicare and Medicaid outpatients are collected by the system?

   a. DEEDS
   b. EMEDS
   c. UACDS
   d. UHDDS

3. Standardizing medical terminology to avoid differences in naming various medical conditions and procedures (such as the synonyms bunionectomy, McBride procedure, and repair of hallus valgus) is one purpose of:

   a. Transaction standards
   b. Content and structure standards
   c. Vocabulary standards
   d. Security standards

4. Patient care managers use the data documented in the health record to:

   a. Evaluate patterns and trends of patient care
   b. Provide direct patient care
   c. Generate patient bills and third-party payer claims for reimbursement
   d. Determine the extent and effects of occupational hazards

5. The active storage area for medical records at Community Hospital is almost filled. To create more space in the storage area, which of the following should be done?

   a. Discard the oldest records
   b. Purge oldest records to another location
   c. Remove nursing notes from the oldest records
   d. Remove the file folders from all the records

6. As part of the initiative to improve data integrity, the Data Quality Committee conducted an inventory of all of the hospital's databases. The review showed more than 70 percent of the identified databases did not have data dictionaries. Given this data, what should be the committee's first action?

   a. Disregard the data.

   b. Establish a data dictionary policy with associated standards.

   c. Develop an in-service training program on data dictionary use.

   d. Distribute a memorandum to all department heads on the value of a data dictionary.

7. Community Hospital has more than 100 clinical databases. The Data Quality Committee is studying the comparability among the databases. The data elements and data definitions are catalogued for each database. What would be the next logical step to determine the degree of data comparability among the databases?

   a. Identify the operating system for each database to determine if they are similar to each other

   b. Select a representative set of data elements and track these across the databases to identify consistencies and differences.

   c. Identify the network capability of each of the databases so that data can be exchanged.

   d. Determine the volume and type of data stored within each database so that a data repository can be developed of similar data.

8. A new HIM director has been asked by the hospital CIO to ensure data content standards are identified, understood, implemented, and managed for the hospital's planned EHR system. Which of the following should be the HIM director's first step in carrying out this responsibility?

   a. Call the EHR vendor and ask to review the system's data dictionary.

   b. Identify data content requirements for all areas of the organization.

   c. Call a meeting of all department directors to get their input.

   d. Contact CMS to determine what data sets are required to be collected.

9. At admission, Mrs. Smith's date of birth is recorded as 3/25/1948. An audit of the electronic health record system discovers that the numbers in the date of birth are transposed in different health record reports. This situation reflects a problem in:

   a. Data comprehensiveness

   b. Data consistency

   c. Data currency

   d. Data granularity

10. A family practitioner requests the opinion of a physician specialist who reviews the patient's health record and examines the patient. The physician specialist would record findings, impressions, and recommendations in what type of report?

    a. Consultation

    b. Medical history

    c. Physical examination

    d. Progress notes

11. Which of the following is a key characteristic of the problem-oriented health record?

    a. Uses an itemized list of the patient's past and present medical problems

    b. Uses laboratory reports and other diagnostic tools to determine medical problems

    c. Allows all providers to document in the health record

    d. Provides electronic documentation in the health record

12. Based on the payment percentages provided in this table, which payer contributes most to the hospital's overall payments?

Payer	Charges	Payments	Adjustment	Charges	Payments	Adjustments
BC/BS	$450,000	$360,000	$90,000	23%	31%	12%
Commercial	$250,000	$200,000	$50,000	13%	17%	6%
Medicaid	$350,000	$75,000	$275,000	18%	6%	36%
Medicare	$750,000	$495,000	$255,000	39%	42%	33%
TRICARE	$150,000	$50,000	$100,000	7%	4%	13%
Total	$1,950,000	$1,180,000	$770,000	100%	100%	100%

    a. BC/BS

    b. Commercial

    c. Medicare

    d. TRICARE

13. Which of the following is true regarding the reporting of communicable diseases?

    a. They must be reported by the patient to the health department.

    b. The diseases to be reported are established by state law.

    c. The diseases to be reported are established by HIPAA.

    d. They are never reported because it would violate the patient's privacy.

14. Data that are collected on large populations of individuals and stored in databases are referred to as:

    a. Statistics

    b. Information

    c. Aggregate data

    d. Standard

15. A health data analyst has been asked to compile a report of the percentage of patients who had a baseline partial thromboplastin time (PTT) performed prior to receiving heparin. What clinical reports in the health record would the health data analyst need to consult in order to prepare this report?

    a. Physician progress notes and medication record

    b. Medication record and clinical laboratory reports

    c. Nursing and physician progress notes

    d. Physician orders and laboratory reports

16. Community Hospital wants to compare its hospital-acquired urinary tract infection (UTI) rate for Medicare patients with the national average. The hospital is using the MEDPAR database for its comparison. The MEDPAR database contains 13,000,000 discharges. 200,000 of these individuals were admitted with a principal diagnosis of UTI; another 300,000 were admitted with a principal diagnosis of infectious disease, and 700,000 had a diagnosis of hypertension. Given this information, which of the following would provide the best comparison data for Community Hospital?

    a. All individuals in the MEDPAR database

    b. All individuals in the MEDPAR database except those admitted with a principal diagnosis of UTI

    c. All individuals in the MEDPAR database except those admitted with a principal diagnosis of UTI or infectious disease

    d. All individuals in the MEDPAR database except those admitted with a diagnosis of hypertension

17. A health data analyst has been asked to compile a listing of daily blood pressure readings for patients with a diagnosis of hypertension that were treated on the medicine unit within a two-week period. What clinical report would be the best source to gather this information?

    a. Admission record

    b. Initial nursing assessment record

    c. Physician progress notes

    d. Vital signs record

18. Given the numbers 47, 20, 11, 33, 30, 30, 35, and 50, what is the median?

    a. 30
    b. 32
    c. 31.5
    d. 35

19. What is (are) the format problem(s) with the following table?

Community Hospital Admissions by Sex, 20XX		
Male	3,546	42.4
Female	4,825	57.6
Total	8,371	100

    a. Variable names are missing

    b. Title of the table is missing

    c. Column headings are missing

    d. Column totals are inaccurate

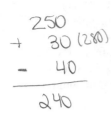

250
+ 30 (280)
- 40
_____
240

9/600

20. Community Hospital had 250 patients in the hospital at midnight on May 1. The hospital admitted 30 patients on May 2. The hospital discharged 40 patients, including deaths, on May 2. Two patients were both admitted and discharged on May 2. What was the total number of inpatient service days for May 2?

   a. 240
   b. 242
   c. 280
   d. 320

21. An example of data collected by the Joint Commission for the ORYX initiatives is:

   a. Intrahospital mortality data
   b. Financial data
   c. Health plan performance data
   d. Patient demographic data

22. Community Hospital HIM department conducted a random sample of 600 health records to determine the rate of filing accuracy. Nine misfiles were identified. Which of the following percentages represents the filing accuracy at Community Hospital?

   a. 15%
   b. 34%
   c. 66.7%
   d. 98.5%

23. Which of the following numbering systems is best for maintaining the encounters of a patient together?

   a. Unit
   b. Serial-unit
   c. Serial
   d. Alphabetical

24. A critical element of data retrieval planning is designing a:

   a. Clinical data repository
   b. Controlled vocabulary
   c. Screen layout
   d. Source systems

25. Which of the following is considered the authoritative key in locating a health record?

   a. Disease index
   b. Master patient index
   c. Patient directory
   d. Patient registry

26. The paper-based health record format that organizes all forms in chronological order is known as a(n):

    a. Problem-oriented health record

    b. Integrated health record

    c. Patient-oriented health record

    d. Source-oriented health record

27. Which of the following is a retention concern with electronic health records?

    a. Durability

    b. Hardware obsolescence

    c. Storage space

    d. Statute of limitations

28. Which of the following lists of names is in correct order for alphabetical filing?

    a. Smith, Carl J.
       Smith, Mary A.
       Smith, Paul M.
       Smith, Thomas

    b. Carl J. Smith
       Mary A. Smith
       Paul M. Smith
       Thomas Smith

    c. Smith, A. Mary
       Smith, J. Carl
       Smith, M. Paul
       Smith, Thomas

    d. Smith, Thomas
       Smith, Carl J.
       Smith, Mary A.
       Smith, Paul M.

29. The RHIT supervisor for the filing and retrieval section of Community Clinic is developing a staffing schedule for the year. The clinic is open 260 days per year and has an average of 500 clinic visits per day. The standard for filing records is 50 records per hour. The standard for retrieval of records is 40 records per hour. Given these standards, how many filing hours will be required daily to retrieve and file records for each clinic day?

    a. 10 hours/day

    b. 11.11 hours/day

    c. 12.5 hours/day

    d. 22.5 hours/day

30. A HIM department is projecting workforce needs for its document scanning process. The intent of the department is to scan patient records at the time of discharge, providing a 24-hour turnaround time. The hospital has an average daily discharge of 120 patients and each patient record has an average of 200 pages. Given the benchmarks listed here, what is the least amount of work hours needed each day to meet a 24-hour turnaround time?

National Benchmarks for Document Scanning Processes	
Function	Expectations per Worked Hour
Prepping	340–500 images
Scanning	1,200–2,400 images
Quality Control	1,600–2,000 images
Indexing	600–800 images

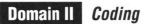

 a. 100 hours
 b. 146 hours
 c. 1,000 hours
 d. 3,740 hours

Domain II *Coding*

31. Which of the following provides a means to record information about patients treated for substance abuse and mental disorders?

 a. Current Procedural Terminology
 b. *Diagnostic and Statistical Manual of Mental Disorders, Fourth Revision*
 c. *International Classification of Diseases, Ninth Revision, Clinical Modification*
 d. Systematized Nomenclature of Medicine Clinical Terminology

32. The HIM department is developing a system to track coding productivity. The director wants the system to track the productivity of each coder by productive hours worked per day, medical record ID, type of records coded and other data, and to provide weekly productivity reports and analyses. Which of the following tools would be best to use for this purpose?

 a. Database management system
 b. Paper log book
 c. Spreadsheet
 d. Word-processing documents

33. Which of the following statements does *not* apply to ICD-9-CM?

 a. It can be used as the basis for epidemiological research.
 b. It can be used in the evaluation of medical care planning for healthcare delivery systems.
 c. It can be used to facilitate data storage and retrieval.
 d. It can be used to collect data about nursing care.

34. Which of the following elements of coding quality represent the degree to which the codes capture all the diagnoses and procedures documented in the patient's health record?

    a. Reliability

    b. Validity

    c. Completeness

    d. Timeliness

35. All of the following are functions of the Outpatient Code Editor, *except*:

    a. Evaluate the relationship between CPT codes on the bill

    b. Control improper coding

    c. Identify unbundling of codes

    d. Identify cases that don't meet medical necessity

36. A patient is admitted for the treatment of dehydration secondary to chemotherapy for primary liver cancer. Which of the following should be sequenced as the principal diagnosis?

    a. Liver carcinoma

    b. Chemotherapy

    c. Dehydration

    d. Complication of chemotherapy

37. The APC payment system is based on what coding system?

    a. CPT/HCPCS codes

    b. ICD-9-CM diagnosis and procedure codes

    c. CPT and ICD-9-CM procedure codes

    d. Only CPT codes

38. A patient was diagnosed with L4-5 lumbar neuropathy and discogenic pain. The patient underwent an intradiscal electrothermal annuloplasty (IDET) in the radiology suite. What ICD-9-CM procedure code is used?

    a. 721.42, Spondylosis with myelopathy, lumbar region

    b. 722.10, Displacement of lumbar intervertebral disc without myelopathy

    c. 80.59, Other destruction of intervertebral disc

    d. 338.22, Chronic post-thoracotomy pain

39. A patient was seen in the emergency department for chest pain. It was suspected that the patient may have gastroesophageal reflux disease (GERD). The final diagnosis was "Rule out GERD." The correct ICD-9-CM diagnosis code is:

    a. V71.7, Observation for suspected cardiovascular disease

    b. 789.01, Abdominal pain, right upper quadrant

    c. 530.81, Esophageal reflux

    d. 786.50, Unspecified chest pain

40. Coding accuracy is best determined by:

    a. A predefined audit process

    b. Medicare Conditions of Participation

    c. Payer audits

    d. Joint Commission Standards for Accreditation

41. Carcinoma of multiple overlapping sites of the bladder. Diagnostic cystoscopy and transurethral fulguration of bladder lesions (1.9 cm, 6.0 cm) are undertaken. Which of the following CPT codes would be most appropriate?

52000	Cystourethroscopy
52224	Cystourethroscopy with fulguration (including cryosurgery or laser surgery) or treatment of minor (less than 0.5 cm) lesion(s) with or without biopsy
52234	Cystourethroscopy with fulguration (including cryosurgery or laser surgery and/or resection of; small bladder tumor(s) (0.5 cm to 2.0 cm)
52235	Cystourethroscopy with fulguration (including cryosurgery or laser surgery) and/or resection of; medium bladder tumor(s) (2.0 cm to 5.0 cm)
52240	Cystourethroscopy with fulguration (including cryosurgery or laser surgery) and/or resection of; large bladder tumor(s)

    a. 52234, 52240

    b. 52235

    c. 52240

    d. 52000, 52234, 52240

42. A laparoscopic tubal ligation is undertaken. Which of the following is the correct CPT code assignment?

49320	Laparoscopy, abdomen, peritoneum, and omentum, diagnostic, with or without collection of specimen(s) by brushing or washing (separate procedure)
58662	Laparoscopy, surgical; with fulguration or excision of lesions of the ovary, pelvic viscera, or peritoneal surface by any method
58670	Laparoscopy, surgical; with fulguration of oviducts (with or without transection)
58671	Laparoscopy, surgical; with occlusions of oviducts by device (eg, band, clip, or Falope ring)

    a. 49320, 58662

    b. 58670

    c. 58671

    d. 49320

43. A patient had a placenta previa with delivery of twins. The patient had two prior cesarean sections. This was an emergent C-section due to hemorrhage. The appropriate principal diagnosis would be:

    a. Normal delivery

    b. Placenta previa

    c. Twin gestation

    d. Vaginal hemorrhage

44. When coding a benign neoplasm of skin of the eyelid, which of the following codes should be used?

216	Benign neoplasm of skin
	Includes:
	Blue nevus
	Dermatofibroma
	Hydrocystoma
	Pigmented nevus
	Syringoadenoma
	Syringoma
	Excludes:
	Skin of genital organs (221.0–222.9)
216.0	Skin of lip
	Excludes:
	Vermilion border of lip (210.0)
216.1	Eyelid, including canthus
	Excludes:
	Cartilage of eyelid (215.0)

a. 216

b. 210.0

c. 215.0

d. 216.1

45. In CPT, if a patient has two lacerations of the arm that are repaired with simple closures, which of the following would apply for correct coding?

a. Two CPT codes, one for each laceration

b. One CPT code for the largest laceration

c. One CPT code, adding the lengths of the lacerations together

d. One CPT code for the most complex closure

46. Carolyn works as a coder in a hospital inpatient department. She sees a lab report in a patient's health record that is positive for staph infection. However, there is no mention of staph in the physician's documentation. What should Carolyn do?

a. Tell her supervisor

b. Query the physician

c. Assign a code for the staph infection

d. Put a note in the chart

47. To clarify documentation, the preferred method of contact between a coder and a physician is:

a. Telephone conversation

b. E-mail transmission

c. Fax transmission

d. Face-to-face communication

48. A skin lesion was removed from a patient's cheek in the dermatologist's office. The dermatologist documents skin lesion, probable basal cell carcinoma. Which of the following actions should the coding professional do to code this encounter?

    a. Code skin lesion
    b. Code benign skin lesion
    c. Code basal cell carcinoma
    d. Query the dermatologist

49. The patient was admitted to the hospital for treatment of a myocardial infarction (heart attack). A bypass procedure was performed on day 2. On day 4, the patient was diagnosed with sepsis, which was not present on admission. Sepsis is a major complication. Based solely on this information, which of the following is the correct MS-DRG assignment for this case?

    a. 235, Coronary bypass w/o cardiac cath w MCC
    b. 236, Coronary bypass w/o cardiac cath w/o MCC
    c. 280, Acute myocardial infarction, discharged alive w MCC
    d. 282, Acute myocardial infarction, discharged alive w/o cc/MCC

50. To use a data element for aggregation and reporting, that data element must be:

    a. Abstracted or indexed
    b. Searched
    c. Subject to case finding
    d. Registered

51. Which of the following record types is most likely to impair an experienced coder's productivity?

    a. 100% EHR
    b. 100% paper record
    c. Source-oriented record
    d. Hybrid record

52. Continuing coding education is required for:

    a. Credentialed coders
    b. Inpatient coders
    c. All coders
    d. Inpatient and ambulatory surgery coders

53. An alternative to the retrospective coding model is the _____ coding model in which records are coded while the patient is still an inpatient in the hospital.

    a. Prospective
    b. Analytical
    c. Concurrent
    d. Auxiliary

54. An inpatient, acute-care coder must follow official ICD-9-CM coding guidelines established by the:

    a. American Health Information Management Association

    b. American Medical Association

    (c.) Centers for Medicare and Medicaid Services

    d. Cooperating Parties

55. A patient was admitted to the hospital with symptoms of a stroke and secondary diagnoses of COPD and hypertension. The patient was subsequently discharged from the hospital with a principal diagnosis of cerebral vascular accident and secondary diagnoses of catheter-associated urinary tract infection, COPD, and hypertension. Which of the following diagnoses should not be reported as POA?

    (a.) Catheter-associated urinary tract infection

    b. Cerebral vascular accident

    c. COPD

    d. Hypertension

56. The first step in an inpatient record review is to verify correct assignment of the:

    a. Record sample

    b. Coding procedures

    (c.) Principal diagnosis

    d. DRG

57. A patient was admitted to the hospital on September 15, 2011, and discharged on October 5, 2011. To code this record correctly, the coder must use the version of ICD-9-CM updated on:

    a. January 1, 2011

    b. April 1, 2011

    (c.) October 1, 2011

    d. October 1, 2012

Domain III *Compliance*

58. To comply with the Joint Commission standards, the HIM director wants to be sure that history and physical examinations are documented in the patient's health record no later than 24 hours after admission. Which of the following would be the best way to ensure the completeness of the health record?

    a. Retrospectively review each patient's medical record to make sure that history and physicals are present.

    b. Review each patient's medical record concurrently to make sure that history and physicals are present.

    c. Establish a process to review medical records immediately on discharge.

    d. Write a memorandum to all physicians relating the Joint Commission requirements for documenting history and physical examinations.

59. Local coverage determinations (LCD) describe when and under what circumstances which of the following is met:

    a. Proper administration of benefits

    b. MACs

    c. NCDs

    d. Medical necessity

60. What factor is medical necessity based on?

    a. The beneficial effects of a service for the patient's physical needs and quality of life

    b. The cost of a service compared with the beneficial effects on the patient's health

    c. The availability of a service at the facility

    d. The reimbursement available for a given service

61. The HIM director is having difficulty with the emergency services on-call physicians completing their health records. Three deficiency notices are sent to the physicians including an initial notice, a second reminder, and a final notification. Which of the following would be the best first step in trying to rectify the current situation?

    a. Routinely send out a fourth notice.

    b. Post the hospital policy in the emergency department.

    c. Consult with the physician in charge of the on-call doctors for suggestions on how to improve response to the current notices.

    d. Call the Joint Commission.

62. Which of the following are basic functions of the utilization management process?

    a. Preadmission review, claims management, and retrospective review

    b. Discharge planning, review for potentially compensable events, and loss prevention

    c. Discharge planning, retrospective review, and preadmission review

    d. Retrospective review, discharge planning, and review for potentially compensable events

63. In developing a monitoring program for coding compliance, which of the following should be regularly audited?

    a. ICD-9-CM and CPT coding

    b. CPT/HCPCS and LOINC coding

    c. ICD-9-CM and SNOMED coding

    d. CPT/HCPCS and SNOMED coding

64. Access to reports based on protected health information within a healthcare facility should be limited to employees who have a:

    a. Report development program

    b. Password

    c. Signed confidentiality agreement

    d. Legitimate need for access

65. In developing an internal coding audit review program, which of the following would be risk areas that should be targeted for audit?

    a. Admission diagnosis and complaints

    b. Chargemaster description

    c. Clinical laboratory results

    d. Radiology orders

66. Which of the following practices is *not* an appropriate coding compliance activity?

    a. Reviewing all rejected claims

    b. Developing procedures for identifying coding errors

    c. Providing a financial incentive for coding claims improperly

    d. Coding diagnoses only when all applicable information is documented in the health record

67. In performing a coding audit, a health record technician discovers that an inpatient coder is assigning diagnosis and procedure codes specifically for the purpose of obtaining a higher level of reimbursement. The coder believes that this practice is helping the hospital in increasing revenue. Which of the following should be done in this case?

    a. Compliment the coder for taking initiative in helping the hospital

    b. Report the coder to the FBI for coding fraud

    c. Counsel the coder and stop the practice immediately

    d. Provide the coder with incentive pay for her actions

68. If a physician does not provide a diagnosis to justify the medical necessity of a service, the provider may obtain payment from the patient:

    a. For the balance due after Medicare has paid

    b. Only if both Medicare and any supplemental insurance have been billed and settled

    c. Never. Providers may never bill Medicare patients for amounts unpaid by Medicare

    d. Only if a properly executed ABN was obtained before the service was provided

69. The utilization manager's role is essential to:

    a. Capture all relevant charges for the patient's account

    b. Verify the patient actually has insurance

    c. Prevent denials for inappropriate levels of service

    d. Analyze the estimate of benefits (EOBs) received

70. The goal of coding compliance programs is to prevent:

    a. Accusations of fraud and abuse

    b. Delays in claims processing

    c. Billing errors

    d. Inaccurate code assignments

71. Which of the following is the approved method for implementing an organization's formal position?

    a. Hierarchy chart

    b. Organizational chart

    c. Policy

    d. Procedure

72. A health record with deficiencies that is not complete within the timeframe specified in the medical staff rules and regulations is called a(n):

    a. Suspended record

    b. Delinquent record

    c. Pending record

    d. Illegal record

73. Which of the following statements is true regarding HIPAA security?

    a. All institutions must implement the same security measures

    b. Institutions are allowed flexibility in the way they implement HIPAA standards

    c. All institutions must implement all HIPAA implementation specifications

    d. A security risk assessment must be performed every year

74. If the coder misrepresents the patient's clinical picture through intentional incorrect coding or the omission or addition of diagnosis or procedure codes, this would be an example of:

    a. Healthcare fraud

    b. Payment optimization

    c. Payment reduction

    d. Healthcare creativity

75. How do accreditation organizations such as the Joint Commission use the health record?

    a. To serve as a source for case study information

    b. To determine whether the documentation supports the provider's claim for reimbursement

    c. To provide healthcare services

    d. To determine whether standards of care are being met

76. Valley High, a skilled nursing facility, wants to become certified to take part in federal government reimbursement programs such as Medicare and Medicaid. What standards must the facility meet to become certified for these programs?

    a. Joint Commission Accreditation Standards

    b. National Commission on Correctional Health Care

    c. Conditions of Participation

    d. Outcomes and Assessment Information Set

77. Which of the following specialized patient assessment tools must be used by Medicare-certified home care providers?

    a. Patient assessment instrument

    b. Minimum data set for long-term care

    c. Resident assessment protocol

    d. Outcomes and Assessment Information Set

78. Before healthcare organizations can provide services, they usually must obtain _____ by government entities such as the state or county in which they are located.

    a. Accreditation

    b. Certification

    c. Licensure

    d. Permission

79. The release of information function requires the HIM professional to have knowledge of:

    a. Clinical coding principals

    b. Database development

    c. Federal and state confidentiality laws

    d. Human resource management

80. A tool that identifies when a user logs in and out, what actions he or she takes, and more is called a(n):

    a. Audit trail

    b. Facility access control

    c. Forensics

    d. Security management plan

81. This database maintains reports on medical malpractice settlements, clinical privilege actions, and professional society membership actions against licensed healthcare providers.

    a. National Practitioners Data Bank

    b. National Physician Database

    c. Healthcare Integrity and Protection Data Bank

    d. Healthcare Security of Physicians Data Bank

7:39

Domain IV *Information Technology*

82. When data has been lost in an electronic health record, which action is taken to remedy this problem?

    a. Data integrity

    b. Data recovery

    c. Firewall

    d. Audit trail

83. Which of the following is used to support the work of professionals engaged in the design, diagnosis, or evaluation of complex situations requiring special knowledge in a limited area?

    a. Decision support system

    b. Executive information system

    c. Expert system

    d. Management information system

84. The HIM and IT departments are working together to justify additional employee password training. The additional training would cost approximately $100,000 with the expectation that password calls to the IT help desk will be reduced by 20 percent. The IT department has done a cost analysis of help desk calls solving password issues. Given this data and approximately 40 password calls per day, can the cost of the additional training be justified?

Costs Associated with Each IT Help Desk Call to Resolve Password Issues	
Personnel	**Cost**
User's time—30 minutes	$15
Telephone cost—30 minutes	$2
Call Desk time—30 minutes	$16
Call Desk IS facilities time	$17
Total	$50

    a. Training will provide $146,000 savings in help desk support and can be justified.

    b. The results of training will provide $365,000 savings in help desk support and can be justified.

    c. The cost of training will be recouped in less than half a year and can be justified.

    d. The cost of training is not justified because qualitative results cannot be measured to calculate a return on investment.

85. The following descriptors about the data element ADMISSION_DATE are included in a data dictionary: definition: date patient admitted to the hospital; data type: date; field length: 15; required field: yes; default value: none; template: none. For this data element, data integrity would be better assured if:

    a. A template was defined

    b. The data type was numeric

    c. The field was not required

    d. The field length was longer

86. Which of the following would be used to control user access in an electronic health record?

    a. Data definition

    b. Relational database

    c. Database management system

    d. Data mining

87. Which of the following is *not* an advantage offered by computer-based clinical decision support tools?

    a. Give physicians instant access to pharmaceutical formularies, referral databases, and reference literature.

    b. Review structured electronic data and alert practitioners to out-of-range laboratory values or dangerous trends.

    c. Help support physicians as they consider diagnostic and treatment alternatives by recalling relevant diagnostic criteria and treatment options on the basis of data in the health record.

    d. Automatically transcribes medical reports.

88. Which of the following best represents the definition of the term *data*?

    a. Patient's laboratory value is 50.

    b. Patient's SGOT is higher than 50 and outside of normal limits.

    c. Patient's resting heart beat is 70, which is within normal range.

    d. Patient's laboratory value is consistent with liver disease.

89. In designing an input screen for an EHR, which of the following would be best to capture discrete data?

    a. Drop-down menus

    b. Speech recognition

    c. Natural language processing

    d. Document imaging

90. A software interface is a:

    a. Device to enter data

    b. Protocol for describing data

    c. Program to exchange data

    d. Standard vocabulary

91. When a hospital uses many different vendors to support its information system needs, the information technology strategy being used is called:

    a. Best of breed

    b. Best of fit

    c. Hospital information system

    d. Legacy architecture

92. Before purchasing an EHR system, a clinical office practice should consult which of the following to ensure the system meets HL7 standards for EHR system functionality?

    a. Certification Commission on Health Information Technology (CCHIT)

    b. Health Information Exchange (HIE)

    c. Centers for Medicare and Medicaid Services (CMS)

    d. National Committee on Vital and Health Statistics (NCVHS)

93. A hospital HIM department wants to purchase an electronic system that records the location of health records removed from the filing system and documents the date of their return to the HIM department. Which of the following electronic systems would fulfill this purpose?

    a. Chart deficiency system

    b. Chart tracking system

    c. Chart abstracting system

    d. Chart encoder

94. Which of the following computer architectures would be best for implementing an EHR for a healthcare system that needs to transmit data to its various campuses that are located across a wide geographic area?

    a. Client/server

    b. Local area network

    c. Wide area network

    d. Wireless network

95. An employee accesses PHI on a computer system that does not relate to her job functions. What security mechanism should have been implemented to minimize this security breach?

    a. Access controls

    b. Audit controls

    c. Contingency controls

    d. Security incident controls

96. Which of the following is the traditional manner of planning and implementing an information system?

    a. CPRI

    b. UML

    c. Database management

    d. SDLC

97. Which of the following is defined as an organized collection of data?

    a. Information

    b. Database

    c. DBMS

    d. Spreadsheet

98. Which of the following is *not* true about a primary key in a database table?

    a. Usually a unique number

    b. Does not change in value

    c. Dependent on the data in the table

    d. Uniquely identifies each row in a table

99. Which of the following allows corporations to supply Internet services over their LANs?

   a. Extranet

   b. Intranet

   c. Internet

   d. WAN

Domain V *Quality*

100. Which tool is used to display performance data over time?

   a. Status process control chart

   b. Run chart

   c. Benchmark

   d. Time ladder

101. The organization that coordinates the collection of performance data for managed care plans is the:

   a. Joint Commission

   b. Centers for Medicare and Medicaid Services

   c. National Committee on Vital and Health Statistics

   d. National Committee for Quality Assurance

102. Problems in patient care and other areas of the healthcare organization are usually symptoms inherent in a(n):

   a. Infrastructure

   b. Output

   c. Principle

   d. System

103. The Leapfrog Group seeks to voluntarily collect data from hospitals about:

   a. The aging healthcare population

   b. Financial costs

   c. Medical errors

   d. Communicable diseases

104. Which of the following statements represents a barrier to implementing performance improvement?

   a. Management demonstrates a high and visible commitment to improvement.

   b. Improvement must be based on good data.

   c. Problems must be viewed as opportunities for improvement.

   d. Employees should not be notified of the change in advance.

105. As part of Community Hospital's organization-wide quality improvement initiative, the HIM director is establishing benchmarks for all of the divisions within the HIM department. The following table shows sample productivity benchmarks for record assembly the director found through a literature search. Given this information, how should the director proceed in establishing benchmarks for the department?

Sample Productivity Benchmarks			
Productivity benchmarks	Per Hour		
Function	Low	Average	High
Assembly (charts per hour)			
Inpatient		8	20
Observation/outpatient surgery/newborn/maternity	5	14	60
Other outpatient		20	120

a. Use the average benchmark example as a beginning point for implementation.

b. Use the low benchmark example as a beginning point for implementation.

c. Determine whether the source of the benchmark data is from a comparable institution.

d. Contact the hospital statistician to determine whether the data are relevant.

106. A quality goal for the hospital is that 98 percent of the heart attack patients receive aspirin within 24 hours of arrival at the hospital. In conducting an audit of heart attack patients, the data showed that 94 percent of the patients received aspirin within 24 hours of arriving at the hospital. Given this data, which of the following actions would be best?

a. Alert the Joint Commission that the hospital has not met its quality goal.

b. Determine whether there was a medical or other reason why patients were not given aspirin.

c. Institute an in-service training program for clinical staff on the importance of administering aspirin within 24 hours.

d. Determine which physicians did not order aspirin.

107. The hospital's Performance Improvement Council has compiled the following data on the volume of procedures performed during 2011. Given this data, which procedures should the council scrutinize in evaluating performance?

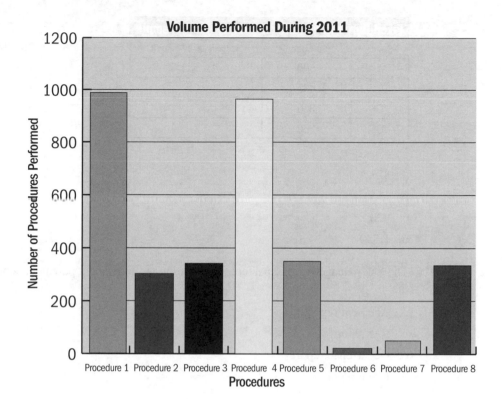

Volume Performed During 2011

a. Procedures 1, 4

b. Procedures 2, 3, 5

c. Procedures 6, 7

d. Procedures 1, 4, 6, 7

108. A member of the hospital's documentation improvement team consistently interrupts others during team meetings. This practice hinders the efficiency of the team. Which of the following would be the best action to take to remedy this situation?

a. Reprimand the offender.

b. Ignore the offender.

c. Develop team ground rules for team communication.

d. Remove the offender from the team.

109. Which of the following is a technique used to generate a large number of creative ideas from a group?

a. Affinity grouping

b. Brainstorming

c. Multivoting technique

d. Nominal group technique

110. A coding supervisor wants to use a fixed percentage random sample of work output to determine coding quality for each coder. Given the work output for each of the four coders shown here, how many total records will be needed for the audit if a 5 percent random sample is used?

Fixed Percentage Random Sample Audit Example		
Coder	Work Output	Records for 5% Audit
A	500	
B	480	
C	300	
D	360	

   a. 82
   b. 156
   c. 820
   d. 1,550

111. The risk manager's principal tool for capturing the facts about potentially compensable events is the:

   a. Accident report
   b. RM report
   c. Occurrence report
   d. Event report

112. Which of the following statements does *not* apply to systems thinking?

   a. Problems in patient care are usually symptoms of shortcomings that are part of a system or process.
   b. Systems thinking is a vital part of performance improvement.
   c. Variations in the way a system works are always caused by factors outside the system.
   d. Every system has inputs and outputs, and the processing of inputs eventually produces outputs.

113. The medical staff is the aggregate of physicians who have been granted permission to provide clinical services in the hospital. What is this permission called?

   a. Medical staff classification
   b. Clinical privileges
   c. Medical staff credentialing
   d. Clinical classification

114. The National Patient Safety Goals score organizations on areas that:

   a. Affect the financial stability of the organization
   b. Commonly lead to overpayment
   c. Affect compliance with state law
   d. Commonly lead to patient injury

115. An audit of the document imaging process reveals that the HIM department staff is scanning 250 pages per hour and indexing 114 pages per hour. If the department is meeting its productivity standard for scanning, but is only meeting 60 percent of the indexing standard, how many more pages per hour must be indexed to meet the indexing standard?

    a. 45.6 pages

    b. 68.4 pages

    c. 76 pages

    d. 190 pages

116. The HIM director has put together a group of department employees to develop coding benchmarks for the number and types of charts to be coded per work hour. The group includes seven employees from the analysis, transcription, release of information, and coding sections. No managers are included on the team because the HIM director wants a bottom-up approach to benchmark development. What fundamental team leadership mistake is the HIM director making with composition of the team?

    a. Too many team members

    b. Unspecific team charge

    c. Insufficient knowledge of team members

    d. Too few team members

117. The quality improvement organizations (QIOs) use peer review, data analysis, and other tools to:

    a. Calculate reimbursement

    b. Identify areas that need improvement

    c. Meet standards for accreditation and licensing

    d. Penalize healthcare organizations

7:56

Domain VI *Legal*

118. Which of the following is an example of an advance directive?

    a. Living will

    b. Authorization to release information

    c. Treatment consent

    d. Patient's rights acknowledgment

119. Community Hospital is terminating its business associate relationship with a medical transcription company. The transcription company has no further need for any identifiable information that it may have obtained in the course of its business with the hospital. The CFO of the hospital believes that to be HIPAA compliant all that is necessary is for the termination to be in a formal letter signed by the CEO. In this case, how should the director of HIM advise the CFO?

    a. Confirm that a formal letter of termination meets HIPAA requirements and no further action is required.

    b. Confirm that a formal letter of termination meets HIPAA requirements and no further action is required except that the termination notice needs to be retained for seven years.

    c. Confirm that a formal letter of termination is required and that the transcription company must provide the hospital with a certification that all PHI that it had in its possession has been destroyed or returned.

    d. Inform the CFO that business associate agreements cannot be terminated.

120. The Medical Record Committee is reviewing the privacy policies for a large outpatient clinic. One of the members of the committee remarks that he feels that the clinic's practice of calling out a patient's full name in the waiting room is not in compliance with HIPAA regulations and that only the patient's first name should be used. Other committee members disagree with this assessment. What should the HIM director advise the committee?

    a. HIPAA does not allow a patient's name to be announced in a waiting room.

    b. There is no violation of HIPAA in announcing a patient's name, but the committee may want to consider implementing practices that might reduce this practice.

    c. HIPAA allows only the use of the patient's first name.

    d. HIPAA requires that patients be given numbers and only the number be announced.

121. The Admissions director maintains that a Notice of Privacy Practices must be provided to the patient on each admission. How should the HIM director respond?

    a. Notice of Privacy Practices is required on the first provision of service.

    b. Notice of Privacy Practices is required every time the patient is provided service.

    c. Notice of Privacy Practices is only required for inpatient admissions.

    d. Notice of Privacy Practices is required on the first inpatient admission but for every outpatient encounter.

122. A hospital receives a valid request from a patient for copies of her medical records. The HIM clerk who is preparing the records removes copies of the patient's records from another hospital where the patient was previously treated. According to HIPAA regulations, was this action correct?

    a. Yes; HIPAA only requires that current records be produced for the patient.

    b. Yes; this is hospital policy for which HIPAA has no control.

    c. No; the records from the previous hospital are considered to be included in the designated record set and should be given to the patient.

    d. No; the records from the previous hospital are not included in the designated record set but should be released anyway.

123. A patient requests copies of her medical records on CD. When the patient goes home, she finds that she cannot read the CD on her computer. The patient then requests the hospital to provide the records in paper format. How should the hospital respond?

    a. Provide the records in paper format.

    b. Burn another CD because this is hospital policy.

    c. Provide the patient with both paper and CD copies of the record.

    d. Review the CD copies with the patient on a hospital computer.

124. A patient requests a copy of his medical records. When the request is received, the HIM clerk finds that the records are stored off-site. Which of the following actions must the hospital take to be in compliance with HIPAA regulations?

    a. Provide copies of the records within 15 days.

    b. Provide copies of the records within 30 days.

    c. Provide copies of the records within 45 days.

    d. Provide copies of the records within 60 days.

125. Which of the following definitions best describes the concept of confidentiality?

    a. The right of individuals to control access to their personal health information

    b. The protection of healthcare information from damage, loss, and unauthorized alteration

    c. The expectation that personal information shared by an individual with a healthcare provider during the course of care will be used only for its intended purpose

    d. The expectation that only individuals with the appropriate authority will be allowed to access healthcare information

126. Ted and Mary are the adoptive parents of Susan, a minor. What is the best way for them to obtain a copy of Susan's operative report?

    a. Wait until Susan is 18.

    b. Present an authorization signed by the court that granted the adoption.

    c. Present an authorization signed by Susan's natural (birth) parents.

    d. Present an authorization that at least one of them (Ted or Mary) has signed.

127. A health information technician receives a subpoena *ad testificandum*. To respond to the subpoena, which of the following should the technician do?

    a. Review the subpoena to determine what documents must be produced.

    b. Review the subpoena and notify the hospital administrator.

    c. Review the subpoena and appear at the time and place supplied to give testimony.

    d. Review the subpoena and alert the hospital's risk management department.

128. A medical group practice has contracted with an HIM professional to help define the practice's legal health record. Which of the following should the HIM professional advise be done first for identifying the components of the legal health record?

    a. Develop a list of all data elements referencing patients that are included in both paper and electronic systems of the practice.

    b. Develop a list of statutes, regulations, rules, and guidelines that contain requirements affecting the release of health records.

    c. Perform a quality check on all health record systems in the practice.

    d. Develop a listing and categorize all information requests for health information over the past two years.

129. Hospital physical documents relating to the delivery of patient care such as medical records, x-rays, laboratory reports, and consultation reports are owned:

    a. By the hospital

    b. By the patient

    c. By the attending and consulting physician

    d. Jointly by the hospital, physician, and patient

130. The right of an individual to keep personal health information from being disclosed to anyone is a definition of:

    a. Confidentiality

    b. Privacy

    c. Integrity

    d. Security

131. What types of covered entity health records are subject to the HIPAA privacy regulations?

    a. Only health records in paper format

    b. Only health records in electronic format

    c. Health records in paper or electronic format

    d. Health records in any format

132. The record custodian typically can testify about which of the following when a party in a legal proceeding is attempting to admit a health record as evidence?

    a. Identification of the record as the one subpoenaed

    b. The care provided to the patient

    c. The qualifications of the treating physician

    d. Identification of the standard of care used to treat the patient

133. Which of the following individuals may authorize release of information?

    a. An 86-year-old patient with a diagnosis of advanced dementia

    b. A married 15-year-old father

    c. A 15-year-old minor

    d. The parents of an 18-year-old student

134. On review of the audit trail for an EHR system, the HIM director discovers that a departmental employee who has authorized access to patient records is printing far more records than the average user. In this case, what should the supervisor do?

    a. Reprimand the employee

    b. Fire the employee

    c. Determine what information was printed and why

    d. Revoke the employee's access privileges

Domain VII *Revenue Cycle*

135. Using the charge description master (CDM) to automatically link a service to the appropriate CPT/HCPCS code is referred to as.

    a. Concurrent coding

    b. Hard coding

    c. Official coding

    d. Upcoding

136. From the information provided in this table, what percentage will the facility be paid for procedure 25500?

Billing Number	Status Indicator	CPT/HCPCS	APC
998323	V	99285–25	0612
998323	T	25500	0044
998323	X	72050	0261
998323	S	72128	0283
998323	S	70450	0283

    a. 0%

    b. 50%

    c. 75%

    d. 100%

137. After appropriate diagnostic and procedural codes are assigned, which of the following must be performed for the provider to be reimbursed in a fee-for-service payment arrangement?

    a. Assign a fee to each service from the provider's standard fee schedule

    b. Discount the fee for each service

    c. Determine bundled services

    d. Bill the third-party payer the capitated premium amount

138. Joe Patient was admitted to Community Hospital. Two days later, he was transferred to Big Medical Center for further evaluation and treatment. He was discharged to home after three days. Community Hospital will receive from Medicare:

    a. The full DRG amount, and Big Medical Center will receive a per diem rate for the three-day stay.

    b. A per diem rate for the two-day stay, and Big Medical Center will receive the full DRG payment.

    c. The full DRG amount, and Big Medical Center will bill Community Hospital a per diem rate for the three-day stay.

    d. No payment. Community Hospital must bill Big Medical Center a per diem rate for the two-day stay.

139. The Accounts Not Selected for Billing Report is used to track accounts that are:

    a. Awaiting payment in accounts receivable

    b. In bill hold or in error and awaiting billing

    c. Paid at different rates

    d. Pulled for quality review

140. Which of the following plans reimburses patients up to a specified amount?

    a. Health insurance

    b. Coinsurance

    c. Indemnity

    d. Major medical plan

141. Which of the following terms is used for the amount charged for a medical insurance policy?

    a. Fee schedule

    b. Premium

    c. Claim

    d. Deductible

142. Major medical insurance covers:

    a. Automobile accidents

    b. Ambulatory care

    c. Catastrophic illnesses

    d. Catastrophic illnesses and injuries

143. In processing a bill for healthcare services, which of the following would be excluded under Medicare Part A?

    a. Dental services

    b. Home health services

    c. Hospice services

    d. Hospitalization services

144. Mrs. Smith is a 75-year-old patient who only has Medicare's Part A insurance. Using the following information, how many benefit periods did the patient use during this calendar year?

Date Admitted	Date Discharged
01/01	01/13
03/20	03/30
07/04	11/02
12/01	12/05

    a. One

    b. Two

    c. Three

    (d.) Four

145. Which of the following would be an example of a common form of healthcare fraud and abuse?

    (a.) Refiling claims after denials

    b. Clinical documentation improvement

    c. Billing for services not furnished to patients

    d. Use of a claim scrubber prior to submitting bills

146. An overarching limitation or maximum dollar plan limit on an insurance plan is also known as:

    a. Benefit cap

    b. Formulary

    c. Copayment

    (d.) Limitation

147. In most instances, the "owner" of the Charge Description Master (CDM) in a healthcare facility is the:

    (a.) HIM department

    b. Information Technology department

    c. Finance department

    d. Patient Accounts department

148. A Clinical Documentation Improvement (CDI) program facilitates accurate coding and helps coders avoid:

    a. NCCI edits

    (b.) Upcoding

    c. Coding without a completed face sheet

    d. Assumption coding

149. The deception or misrepresentation by a healthcare provider that may result in a false or fictitious claim for inappropriate payment by Medicare or other insurers for items or services either not rendered or rendered to a lesser extent than described in the claim is:

    a. Healthcare fraud
    b. Optimization
    c. Upcoding
    d. Healthcare abuse

150. A _____ assists in educating medical staff members on documentation needed for accurate billing.

    a. Physician champion
    b. Compliance officer
    c. Chargemaster coordinator
    d. Data monitor

EXAM 2

Domain I Data Analysis and Management

1. Which of the following data sets would be most helpful in developing a hospital trauma data registry?

    a. DEEDS

    b. UACDS

    c. MDS

    d. OASIS

2. Treatment plans and instructions are an example of which of the NHIN dimensions?

    a. Personal health

    b. Healthcare provider

    c. Population health

    d. Payer

3. Community Hospital's HIM department conducted a random sample of 540 health records to determine the rate of filing accuracy. Thirteen misfiles were identified. Which of the following percentages represents the filing accuracy at Community Hospital?

    a. 2.4%

    b. 24.0%

    c. 41.5%

    d. 97.6%

4. Activities of daily living (ADL) are components of:

    a. UACDS

    b. UHDDS

    c. OASIS

    d. ORYX and RAPs

5. Managing an organization's data and those who enter it is an ongoing challenge requiring active administration and oversight. This can be accomplished by the organization through management of which of the following?

    a. Data dictionary

    b. Data warehouse

    c. Data mapping

    d. Data set

6. A consumer nonprofit organization wants to conduct studies on the quality of care provided to Medicare patients in a specific region. A HIT professional has been hired to manage this project. The nonprofit organization asks the HIT professional about the viability of using billing data as the basis for its analysis. Which of the following would *not* be a quality consideration in using billing data?

   a. Accuracy of the data

   b. Consistency of the data

   c. Appropriateness of the data elements

   d. Cost to process the data

7. In a routine health record quantitative analysis review, it was found that a physician dictated a discharge summary on 1/26/2010. Because of unexpected complications, however, the patient was discharged two days after the discharge summary was dictated. What would be the best course of action in this case?

   a. Request that the physician dictate another discharge summary.

   b. Have the record analyst note the date discrepancy.

   c. Request the physician dictate an addendum to the discharge summary.

   d. File the record as complete because the discharge summary includes all of the pertinent patient information.

8. A hospital's electronic health system defines the expected values of the gender data element as female, male, and unknown. This type of specificity is known as:

   a. Data comprehensiveness

   b. Data consistency

   c. Data granularity

   d. Data precision

9. Which of the following documentation must be included in a patient's medical record prior to performing a surgical procedure?

   a. Consent for operative procedure, anesthesia report, surgical report

   b. Consent for operative procedure, history, physical examination

   c. History, physical examination, anesthesia report

   d. Problem list, history, physical examination

10. Which of the following reports includes names of the surgeon and assistants, date, duration, and description of the procedure and any specimens removed?

   a. Operative report

   b. Anesthesia report

   c. Pathology report

   d. Laboratory report

11. The hospital currently has a hybrid health record. Nurses and clinicians are recording bedside documentation electronically in a clinical documentation system, while most other documentation, such as physician progress notes and orders are paper based and stored in a paper medical record. Retrieval of the complete record after discharge is difficult. The HIM director believes that the integrity of the record is at risk since it is harder to control addenda and updates when the record is spread between electronic and paper systems. Furthermore, physicians find it difficult to locate documentation if the patient is readmitted at a later date. Given these circumstances, which of the following should the HIM director implement to alleviate these problems and preserve the efficiencies of an electronic record?

    a. Print out all electronic data post-discharge and file with the rest of the paper record.

    b. Microfilm all electronic data and link to the paper record.

    c. Digitally scan all paper records post-discharge and integrate and index these into the existing digital documentation system.

    d. Digitally scan all paper records.

12. A hospital HIM department wants to move five years of medical records to a remote storage location. The records will be stored in boxes and will be filed on open shelves at the remote location. Which of the following should be done so that record location can be easily identified in the remote storage area?

    a. Provide a unique identifier for each box and prepare a log of the records that is cross-indexed by box identifier.

    b. Prepare a sequential list of all records sent to remote storage.

    c. Provide a unique box identifier and list the records by medical record number on the outside of each box.

    d. File the records in terminal digit order in each box.

13. The HIM department has recently performed an audit of medical records. The audit showed that for the 10,000 records filed there was a 7 percent error rate. Given that the national average cost of each misfile results in a $200 labor cost, what is the labor cost for the department for handling these misfiled records?

    a. $1,400

    b. $14,000

    c. $140,000

    d. $285,714

14. Identify the acute-care report where the following information would be found: "HEENT: Reveals the tympanic membranes, nares, and pharynx to be clear. No obvious head trauma. CHEST: Good bilateral chest sounds."

    a. Discharge summary

    b. Medical history

    c. Medical laboratory report

    d. Physical examination

15. Cancer registries are established by hospitals:

    a. By federal law or state law

    b. Voluntarily or by state law

    c. Voluntarily or by federal law

    d. By mandate from the American College of Surgeons

16. The HIM director is part of the revenue cycle management team. The discharged-not-final-billed days are increasing because discharges are increasing. The number of coding staff is five. In an effort to increase productivity, the HIM director is researching staffing alternatives. With the implementation of an electronic document storage system, telecommuting has been suggested as an alternative. Studies have reported that coding productivity can increase as much as 20 percent with telecommuting. Given that discharges have increased from 100 per day to 144, how many more FTEs would need to be hired if the department went to telecommuting?

    a. 0.5 FTE

    b. 0.75 FTE

    c. 1 FTE

    d. 2 FTEs

17. If an employee produces 2,080 hours of work in the course of a year, how many employees will be required for the coding area if the coding time on average for one record is 30 minutes and there are 12,500 records that must be coded each year?

    a. 3

    b. 6

    c. 36

    d. 69

18. The link that tracks patient, person, or member activity within healthcare organizations and across patient care settings is known as:

    a. The master patient index (MPI)

    b. Benchmarking

    c. Case-mix management

    d. The OIG work plan

19. In addition to case mix, other factors that may influence episode-related data quality include all of the following *except*:

    a. Length of inpatient stay

    b. Health record documentation

    c. Data abstract type

    d. Workflow issues

20. Patient name, zip code, and health record number are typical:

    a. Data fields

    b. Data sources

    c. Aggregate data

    c. Data monitors

21. You are the director of HIM at Community Hospital. One of your physicians has asked you for the total number of appendectomies that he performed at your hospital last year. You will provide the physician with:

    a. Patient-specific data

    b. Aggregate data

    c. Operating room data

    d. Nothing. You cannot obtain this data after the fact

22. Which of the following can assist managers with the tasks of monitoring productivity and forecasting budgets?

    a. Workload statistics

    b. Intermediary bulletins

    c. Revenue codes

    d. Mapping errors

23. Suppose that you want to display the number of deaths due to breast cancer for the years 1998 through 2008. What is the best graphic technique to use?

    a. Table

    b. Histogram

    c. Line graph

    d. Bar chart

24. In May, 270 women were admitted to the obstetrics service. Of these, 263 women delivered; 33 deliveries were by C-section. What is the denominator for calculating the C-section rate?

    a. 33

    b. 263

    c. 270

    d. 296

25. Community Hospital had a total of 3,000 inpatient service days for the month of September. What was the average daily census for the hospital during September?

    a. 10 patients

    b. 96.77 patients

    c. 97 patients

    d. 100 patients

26. Community Hospital discharged 9 patients on April 1. The length of stay for each of the patients was as follows: for patient A, 1 day; for patient B, 5 days; for patient C, 3 days; for patient D, 3 days; for patient E, 8 days; for patient F, 8 days; for patient G, 8 days; for patient H, 9 days; for patient I, 9 days. What was the average length of stay for these nine patients?

    a. 5 days

    b. 6 days

    c. 8 days

    d. 9 days

27. What is the information identifying the patient (such as name, health record number, address, and telephone number) called?

    a. Accession data

    b. Indicator data

    c. Reference data

    d. Demographic data

28. A hospital can monitor its performance under the MS-DRG system by monitoring its:

    a. Accounts receivable

    b. Operating costs

    c. RBRVS payments

    d. Case-mix index

29. AHIMA's retention standards recommend that the master patient index be maintained:

    a. For at least 5 years

    b. For at least 10 years

    c. For at least 25 years

    d. Permanently

30. In designing a paper-based storage system, which of the following should be used if conservation of floor space is the major concern?

    a. Carousel system

    b. Five-drawer filing cabinets

    c. Mobile filing units

    d. Open-shelf filing units

Domain II *Coding*

31. Which of the following elements of coding quality represent consistency of code assignments among different coders?

    a. Reliability

    b. Validity

    c. Completeness

    d. Timeliness

32. Volume 1 of ICD-9-CM contains which one of the following?

    a. Numerical listing of disease codes ranging from 001 to 999.9

    b. Numerical listing of procedure codes ranging from 01 to 99.9

    c. Morphology codes

    d. Alphabetic Index to Diseases

33. Patient accounting is reporting an increase in national coverage decisions (NCDs), and local coverage determinations (LCDs) failed edits in observation accounts. Which of the following departments will be tasked to resolve this issue?

    a. Utilization Management

    b. Patient Access

    c. Health Information Management

    d. Patient Accounts

34. Coding productivity consists of:

    a. Accuracy and volume

    b. Accuracy

    c. Volume

    d. CMI

35. Presentations on complex DRGs should include the etiology and manifestations of conditions, along with:

    a. Symptoms

    b. A review of anatomy and physiology

    c. Related complications

    d. How DRG results are reported

36. Which of the following is *not* one of the purposes of ICD-9-CM?

    a. Classification of morbidity for statistical purposes

    b. Classification of mortality for statistical purposes

    c. Reporting of diagnoses by physicians

    d. Identification of the supplies, products, and services provided to patients

37. All of the following can be used to develop a focused inpatient coding review *except*:

    a. Controversial issues identified in AHA *Coding Clinic*

    b. Recent data quality issues identified by external review agencies

    c. Analysis of comparative data

    d. Top 25 APC groups by volume and charges

38. The staff member who is responsible for evaluating and monitoring education action plans for individual coders within a coding department is the:

    a. Compliance officer

    b. Data quality specialist

    c. Attending physician

    d. Coding manager

39. Which volume of ICD-9-CM contains the numerical listing of codes that represent diseases and injuries?

    a. Volume 1

    b. Volume 2

    c. Volume 3

    d. Volume 4

40. When coding benign neoplasm of the skin, the section noted here directs the coder to:

216	Benign neoplasm of skin
	Includes:
	Blue nevus
	Dermatofibroma
	Hydrocystoma
	Pigmented nevus
	Syringoadenoma
	Syringoma
	Excludes:
	Skin of genital organs (221.0–222.9)
216.0	Skin of lip
	Excludes:
	Vermilion border of lip (210.0)
216.1	Eyelid, including canthus
	Excludes:
	Cartilage of eyelid (215.0)

    a. Use category 216 for syringoma.

    b. Use category 216 for malignant melanoma.

    c. Use category 216 for malignant neoplasm of the bone.

    d. Use category 216 for malignant neoplasm of the skin.

41. A 65-year-old patient is admitted with pain and loosening of a previous total hip arthroplasty. The acetabular component has loosened and become painful. The patient was admitted for revision of the hip replacement. The acetabular component uses a metal-on-metal bearing surface. Which of the following codes would be the appropriate coding for the admission?

996.41	Mechanical loosening of prosthetic joint
996.66	Infection and inflammatory reaction due to internal joint prosthesis
V43.64	Organ or tissue replaced by other means, hip
00.71	Revision hip replacement, acetabular component
00.74	Revision hip replacement bearing surface, metal on polyethylene
00.75	Revision hip replacement bearing surface, metal on metal

    a. 996.41, V43.64, 00.71, 00.75

    b. 996.96, 00.75

    c. 996.41, V43.64, 00.71, 00.74

    d. 996.96, V43.64, 00.71, 00.75

42. The patient was discharged with the following diagnoses: Cerebral occlusion, hemiparesis, asphasia, and hypertension. Which of the following code assignments would be appropriate for this case?

342.90	Hemiparesis affecting unspecified side
342.91	Hemiparesis affecting dominant side
342.92	Hemiparesis affecting nondominant side
434.90	Cerebral artery occlusion unspecified
434.91	Cerebral artery occlusion with infarction
401.0	Malignant hypertension
401.1	Benign hypertension
401.9	Unspecified hypertension
428.0	Congestive heart failure
784.3	Aphasia

   a. 434.91, 342.92, 784.3, 401.1

   b. 434.90, 342.90, 784.3, 401.9

   c. 434.90, 342.91, 784.3, 401.9

   d. 434.90, 342.90, 784.3, 401.0

43. According to CPT, an endoscopy that is undertaken to the level of the midtransverse colon would be coded as a:

   a. Proctosigmoidoscopy

   b. Sigmoidoscopy

   c. Colonoscopy

   d. Proctoscopy

44. Which of the following is on the list of hospital-acquired conditions provision of the inpatient prospective payment system?

   a. Congestive heart failure

   b. Acute myocardial infarction

   c. Pressure ulcers

   d. Diabetic retinopathy

45. A secondary condition that arises during a patient's hospitalization is known by which of the following terms?

   a. Comorbidity

   b. Secondary diagnosis

   c. Complication

   d. Evaluation and management code

46. From the information provided, how many APCs would this patient have?

Billing Number	Status Indicator	CPT/HCPCS	APC
998323	V	99285–25	0612
998323	T	25500	0044
998323	X	72050	0261
998323	S	72128	0283
998323	S	70450	0283

    a. 1

    b. 4

    c. 5

    d. Unable to determine

47. A patient is admitted to the hospital with shortness of breath and congestive heart failure. The patient subsequently develops respiratory failure. The patient undergoes intubation with ventilator management. Which of the following would be the correct sequencing and coding of this case?

    a. Congestive heart failure, respiratory failure, ventilator management, intubation

    b. Respiratory failure, intubation, ventilator management

    c. Respiratory failure, congestive heart failure, intubation, ventilator management

    d. Shortness of breath, congestive heart failure, respiratory failure, ventilator management

48. A physician correctly prescribes Coumadin. The patient takes the Coumadin as prescribed, but develops hematuria as a result of taking the medication. Which of the following is the correct way to code this case?

    a. Poisoning due to Coumadin

    b. Unspecified adverse reaction to Coumadin

    c. Hematuria; poisoning due to Coumadin

    d. Hematuria; adverse reaction to Coumadin

49. In reviewing a patient chart, the coder finds that the patient's chest x-ray is suggestive of chronic obstructive pulmonary disease (COPD). The attending physician mentions the x-ray finding in one progress note, but no medication, treatment, or further evaluation is provided. Which of the following actions should the coder take in this case?

    a. Query the attending physician and ask him to validate the COPD as a diagnosis.

    b. Code the COPD because the documentation substantiates it.

    c. Query the radiologist to determine whether the patient has the COPD.

    d. Assign a code from the abnormal findings to reflect the condition.

50. Placenta previa with delivery of twins. This patient had two prior cesarean sections. She also has a third-degree perineal laceration. This was an emergent C-section due to hemorrhage associated with the placenta previa. The appropriate principal diagnosis would be:

    a. Third-degree perineal laceration

    b. Placenta previa

    c. Twin gestation

    d. Vaginal hemorrhage

51. A patient is admitted to the hospital with abdominal pain. The principal diagnosis is cholecystitis. The patient also has a history of hypertension and diabetes. In the DRG prospective payment system, which of the following would determine the MDC assignment for this patient?

    a. Abdominal pain

    b. Cholecystitis

    c. Hypertension

    d. Diabetes

52. The sum of a hospital's relative DRG weights for a year was 15,192, and the hospital had 10,471 discharges for the year. Given this information, what would be the hospital's case-mix index for that year?

    a. 0.689

    b. 0.689×100

    c. 1.45×100

    d. 1.45

53. Given the information here, which of the following MS-DRGs would have the highest payment?

MS-DRG	MDC	Type	MS-DRG Title	Weight	Discharges	Geometric Mean	Arithmetic Mean
191	04	MED	Chronic obstructive pulmonary disease w CC	0.9628	10	3.7	4.5
192	04	MED	Chronic obstructive pulmonary disease w/o CC/MCC	0.7081	20	3.0	3.5
193	04	MED	Simple pneumonia & pleurisy w MCC	1.4948	10	5.2	6.4
194	04	MED	Simple pneumonia & pleurisy w CC	1.0026	20	4.0	4.8
195	04	MED	Simple pneumonia & pleurisy w/o CC/MCC	0.7037	10	3.0	3.6

    a. 191

    b. 192

    c. 193

    d. 194

54. Which of the following is most likely to be used in performing an outpatient coding review?

    a. OCE

    b. MS-DRG

    c. CMI

    d. MDS

55. Which of the following is a condition that arises during hospitalization?

    a. Case mix

    b. Complication

    c. Comorbidity

    d. Principal diagnosis

56. A HIM department is planning to implement virtual teams for the coding and the data analytics areas. Some in the facility are skeptical of this arrangement, believing that off-site employees cannot be managed. Given this work format, how can the supervisor best gauge productivity of the virtual staff?

    a. Require staff to call in to the office every morning.

    b. Require a daily conference call with all staff.

    c. Set clear goals and productivity standards and see that these are met.

    d. Install camcorders on each team's computer to ensure that they are at their workstations.

57. The following are reporting options to assign POA *except*:

    a. Y—Present at the time of inpatient admission

    b. N—Not present at the time of inpatient admission

    c. E—Exempt from POA reporting

    d. W—Provider is unable to clinically determine whether condition was POA

Domain III *Compliance*

58. In developing an internal coding audit review program, which of the following would be risk areas that should be targeted for audit?

    a. Admission diagnosis and complaints

    b. Chargemaster description and medical necessity

    c. Clinical laboratory results

    d. Radiology orders

59. During a review of documentation practices, the HIM director finds that nurses are routinely using the copy and paste function of the hospital's new EHR system for documenting nursing notes. In some cases nurses are copying and pasting the objective data from the lab system and intake–output records. In other cases the nurses are copying patient's subjective complaints originally documented by another practitioner. Which of the following should the HIM director do to ensure that the nurses are following acceptable documentation practices?

    a. Inform the nurses that copy and paste is not acceptable and to stop this practice immediately.

    b. Determine how many nurses are involved in this practice.

    c. Institute an in-service training session on documentation practices.

    d. Develop policy and procedures related to cutting, copying, and pasting documentation in the EHR system.

60. The OIG states that insufficient or missing documentation and one of the following are responsible for 70 percent of bad claims submitted to Medicare.

    a. Local coverage decisions

    b. Unbundling of procedures

    c. Failure to document medical necessity

    d. Overcoding

61. Which of the following should be *avoided* when designing forms for an electronic document management system (EDMS)?

    a. Quarter-inch border on each side of document without bar code

    b. Mnemonic descriptor used for non-barcode recognition engine

    c. Color borders around the edge of a form

    d. Shading of bars or lines that contain text

62. During an audit of health records, the HIM director finds that transcribed reports are being changed by the author up to a week after initial transcription. The director is concerned that changes occurring this long after transcription jeopardize the legal principle that documentation must occur near the time of the event. To remedy this situation, the HIM director should recommend which of the following?

    a. Immediately stop the practice of changing transcribed reports.

    b. Develop a facility policy that defines the acceptable period of time allowed for a transcribed document to remain in draft form.

    c. Conduct a verification audit.

    d. Alert hospital legal counsel of the practice.

63. In a managed fee-for-service arrangement, which of the following would be used as a cost-control process for inpatient surgical services?

    a. Prospectively precertify the necessity of inpatient services

    b. Determine what services can be bundled

    c. Pay only 80% of the inpatient bill

    d. Require the patient to pay 20% of the inpatient bill

64. Which of the following is the principal goal of internal auditing programs for billing and coding?

    a. Increase revenues

    b. Protect providers from sanctions or fines

    c. Improve patient care

    d. Limit unnecessary changes to the Chargemaster

65. The National Practitioner Data Bank is associated most closely with which hospital function?

    a. Billing

    b. Coding

    c. Credentialing

    d. Surgeries

66. What is the role of the case manager?

    a. Perform retrospective utilization reviews

    b. Implement the prospective payment system for acute care

    c. Coordinate medical care and ensure the necessity of the services provided to beneficiaries

    d. Ensure that the hospital's resources are being used efficiently

67. Precise coding helps to ensure _____ regulatory requirements.

    a. Awareness of

    b. Validation of

    c. Compliance with

    d. Quality standards consistent with

68. Which governmental fraud and abuse effort focused on recouping lost funds for the Medicare program due to inaccurate coding and billing? $188 million were recovered during the first two years of this effort.

    a. Hospital Payment Monitoring Program

    b. OIG Compliance Program Guidance

    c. Operation Restore Trust

    d. Medicare Integrity Program

69. One way for a hospital to demonstrate compliance with OIG guidelines is to:

    a. Designate a privacy officer

    b. Continuously monitor PEPPER reports

    c. Obtain ABNs for all Medicare registrations

    d. Develop, implement, and monitor written policies and procedures

70. Healthcare abuse relates to practices that may result in:

    a. False representation of fact

    b. Failure to disclose a fact

    c. Medically unnecessary services

    d. Altered claim forms

71. The hospital is revising its policy on medical record documentation. Currently, all entries in the medical record must be legible, complete, dated, and signed. The committee chairperson wants to add that, in addition, all entries must have the time noted. However, another clinician suggests that adding the time of notation is difficult and rarely may be correct since personal watches and the hospital clocks may not be coordinated. Another committee member agrees and says that only electronic documentation needs a time stamp. Given this discussion, which of the following might the HIM director suggest?

    a. Suggest that only hospital clock time be noted in clinical documentation.

    b. Suggest that only electronic documentation have time notated.

    c. Inform the committee that according to the Conditions of Participation all documentation must include date and time.

    d. Inform the committee that according to the Conditions of Participation only medication orders must include date and time.

72. Site-of-service documents to help providers develop compliance programs have been published by the:

    a. Joint Commission

    b. American Health Information Management Association (AHIMA)

    c. Office of the Inspector General (OIG)

    d. Centers for Medicare and Medicaid Services (CMS)

73. The document that demonstrates the steps an HIM department is taking to ensure data quality is called the:

    a. Departmental coding compliance manual

    b. Coding standards

    c. Code of conduct

    d. Coding compliance plan

74. Which of the following would be part of the release of information system?

    a. Letter asking for additional information on a patient previously treated at the hospital

    b. Letter notifying individual that the authorization was invalid

    c. Letter notifying physician that he has delinquent medical records

    d. Letter asking physician to clarify primary diagnosis

75. What Joint Commission mandate does the chart location system assist with compliance?

    a. Security

    b. Privacy

    c. Accessibility

    d. Documentation

76. Which of the following can be defined as a voluntary system of institutional review in which a quasi-independent body periodically evaluates the quality of the services provided by healthcare organizations against written criteria?

    a. Accreditation

    b. Standardization

    c. Licensure

    d. Professionalization

77. A hospital CEO wants to organize the organization's policies, procedures, and business expertise to increase overall effectiveness and efficiency. Which of the following systems would be best to accomplish this task?

    a. Data warehouse

    b. Decision support system

    c. Knowledge management system

    d. Management information system

78. Which of the following should be considered *first* when establishing health record retention policies?

    a. State retention requirements

    b. Accreditation standards

    c. AHIMA's retention guidelines

    d. Federal requirements

79. A dietary department donated its old microcomputer to a school. Some old patient data were still on the microcomputer. What controls would have minimized this security breach?

    a. Access controls

    b. Device and media controls

    c. Facility access controls

    d. Workstation controls

80. The first and most fundamental strategy for minimizing security threats is to:

    a. Establish access controls

    b. Implement an employee security awareness program

    c. Establish a security organization

    d. Conduct a risk analysis

81. A coding compliance manager is reviewing a tool that identifies when a user logs in and out, what he or she does, and more. What is the manager reviewing?

    a. Audit trail

    b. Facility access control

    c. Forensics

    d. Security management plan

Domain IV   *Information Technology*

82. A health data analyst has been asked to abstract patient demographic information into an electronic database. Which of the following would the analyst *not* include in the database?

    a. Patient date of birth

    b. Name of next of kin

    c. Date and time of admission

    d. Admitting diagnosis

83. A physician wants an automated system that allows input of signs, symptoms, and results of laboratory tests and provides a list of provisional diagnoses. Which of the following would best meet the physician's needs?

    a. Clinical decision support system

    b. Decision support system

    c. Executive information system

    d. Management information system

84. Which of the following end users would normally use a management information system in their day-to-day work?

    a. Clerical staff

    b. Laboratory technicians

    c. Admissions clerks

    d. Department directors

85. Which of the following would be the best technique to ensure nurses do not omit any essential information on the nursing intake assessment in an EHR?

    a. Provide an input mask for essential data fields.

    b. Make all essential data fields required.

    c. Put validation edits on all essential fields.

    d. Provide sufficient space for all essential fields.

86. Which of the following can be defined as a collection of related components that interact to perform a task to accomplish a goal?

    a. Information

    b. Data

    c. System

    d. Process

87. Which of the following information systems manages the day-to-day operations of a business?

    a. Transaction processing system

    b. Management information system

    c. Decision-processing system

    d. Expert system

88. Which of the following provides organizations with the ability to access data from multiple databases and to combine the results into a single questions-and-reporting interface?

    a. Client–server computer

    b. Data warehouse

    c. Local area network

    d. Internet

89. In hospitals, automated systems for registering patients and tracking their encounters are commonly known as _____ systems.

    a. MIS

    b. CDS

    c. ADT

    d. ABC

90. The following data fields comprise a database table: patient last name, patient first name, street address, city, state, zip code, patient date of birth. Given this information, which of the following is a true statement about maintaining the data integrity of the database table?

    a. Patient last name should be used as the primary key for the table.

    b. Patient date of birth should be used as the primary key for the table.

    c. None of the data fields are adequate to use as a primary key for the table.

    d. Patient last and first name should be used as the primary key for the table.

91. Which of the following would be the best technique to ensure that registration clerks consistently use the correct notation for assigning admission date in an electronic health record?

    a. Make admission date a required field.

    b. Provide a template for entering data in the field.

    c. Make admission date a numeric field.

    d. Provide sufficient space for input of data.

92. Which of the following is used as sketch of the user interface during system development?

    a. Screen prototype

    b. System testing

    c. System debugging

    d. System object

93. Which of the following should be done before implementing a new clinical information system?

    a. Test the system with actual patient data.

    b. Test the system with data supplied by the vendor.

    c. Test the system with test data.

    d. Test the system with training data.

94. Which of the following strategies would be best to ensure that all stakeholders are engaged in the planning and development of an organization EHR system?

    a. Form an EHR steering committee

    b. Put out a press release

    c. Distribute an organization-wide memorandum from the CEO

    d. Put out a notice on the organization's intranet

95. The three elements of a security program are ensuring data availability, protection, and:

    a. Suitability

    b. Integrity

    c. Flexibility

    d. Robustness

96. A coding analyst consistently enters the wrong code for patient gender in the computer billing system. What security measures should be in place to minimize this security breach?

    a. Access controls

    b. Audit trail

    c. Edit checks

    d. Password controls

97. A hospital is planning on allowing coding professionals to work at home. The hospital is in the process of identifying strategies to minimize the security risks associated with this practice. Which of the following would be best to ensure that data breaches are minimized when the home computer is unattended?

    a. User name and password

    b. Automatic session terminations

    c. Cable locks

    d. Encryption

98. In a database the LAST_NAME column in a table would be considered a:

    a. Data element

    b. Record

    c. Primary key

    d. Row

99. An information system that alerts a physician when a laboratory value is outside of the normal range is called a(n):

    a. Clinical decision support system

    b. Enterprise-wide system

    c. Management information system

    d. Transaction processing system

Domain V *Quality*

100. Data collected to evaluate facility performance in designated core measure areas to achieve accreditation is:

    a. HEDIS

    b. ORYX

    c. DEEDS

    d. OASIS

101. Which of the following statements does *not* represent a principle of contemporary performance improvement?

    a. Success must be celebrated to encourage more success.

    b. All systems demonstrate variation.

    c. Performance improvement works by identifying the individuals responsible for quality problems and reprimanding them.

    d. Performance improvement relies on the collection and analysis of data to increase knowledge.

102. The success of organizational efforts at change depends on the:

    a. Organization's culture of shared vision, responsibility, and accountability

    b. Chief executive officer's ability to get the administrative and clinical staff's buy-in for the change

    c. Employees' immediate acceptance of the need for change

    d. Traditional leadership skills of the organization's governing board

103. Which of the following is *not* an example of a private or governmental group focused on quality?

    a. Institute for Healthcare Improvement

    b. Safe Practices for All

    c. Commonwealth Fund

    d. Leapfrog Group

104. The traditional approach to ensuring quality was to view quality as the:

    a. Execution of an activity

    b. Absence of defects

    c. Absence of corrective action

    d. Application of interpersonal skills

105. Two coders have found the same abbreviation on two records. One abbreviation of "O.D." was used on an eye health record to mean "right eye." The other abbreviation on another patient's record was used to mean "overdose" on an abuse record. What data quality component is lacking here?

    a. Timeliness

    b. Completeness

    c. Security

    d. Consistency

106. Performance improvement teams should report on their progress and activities to the organization's Performance Improvement and Patient Safety Council at least:

    a. Weekly

    b. Monthly

    c. Quarterly

    d. Annually

107. The hospital-acquired infection rate for our hospital is 0.2%, whereas the rate at a similar hospital across town is 0.3%. This is an example of:

    a. Benchmark

    b. Check sheet

    c. Data abstract

    d. Run chart

108. The leader of the coding performance improvement team wants all of her team members to clearly understand the coding process. Which of the following would be the best tool for accomplishing this objective?

    a. Flowchart

    b. Force-field analysis

    c. Pareto chart

    d. Scatter diagram

109. The credentialing process of independent practitioners within a healthcare organization must be defined in:

    a. Hospital policies and procedures

    b. Medical staff bylaws

    c. Accreditation regulations

    d. Hospital licensure rules

110. The medical transcription improvement team wants to identify the cause of poor transcription quality. Which of the following tools would best aid the team in identifying the root cause of the problem?

    a. Flowchart

    b. Fishbone diagram

    c. Pareto chart

    d. Scatter diagram

111. Which of the following statements does *not* represent a fundamental principle of performance improvement?

    a. Teamwork is an optional element in performance improvement.

    b. Communication must be open and honest.

    c. Success must be celebrated to encourage more success.

    d. Leaders and employees must know and share the organization's mission and vision.

112. Community Hospital has been collecting quarterly data on the average monthly medical record delinquency rate for the hospital. This graph depicts the trend in the delinquency rate. The hospital has established a 35% benchmark. Given this data, what should the hospital's Performance Improvement Council recommend?

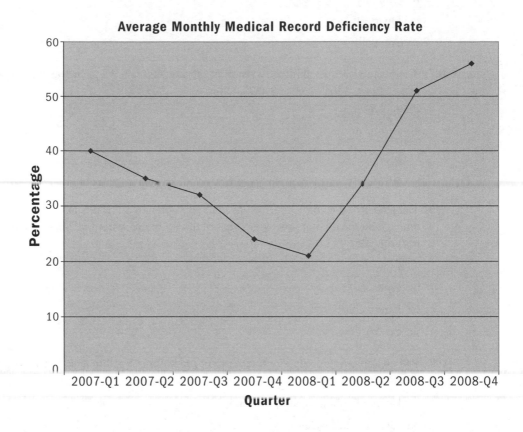

Average Monthly Medical Record Deficiency Rate

a. Maintain tracking the delinquency rate to see if the last two-quarter trend continues.

b. Establish a higher benchmark to accommodate an increase in delinquent records.

c. Further analyze the data to determine why the benchmark is not being met.

d. Take an average of all the data points to arrive at a new benchmark.

113. Which of the following is the goal of the quantitative analysis performed by HIM professionals?

a. Ensuring that the health record is legible

b. Identifying deficiencies early so they can be corrected

c. Verifying that health professionals are providing appropriate care

d. Ensuring bills are correct

114. Which of the following quality indicators measure the things devices or people do?

a. Structure indicators

b. Process indicators

c. Outcome indicators

d. Teamwork indicators

115. An HIM professional is the leader of the quality improvement team. To ensure all team members understand purpose of the team, which of the following actions should be taken?

    a. Develop project definition document

    b. Record minutes of the first team meeting

    c. Develop a mission statement

    d. Develop a Gantt chart

116. An HIM supervisor is revising job descriptions for record scanning positions. These positions have been in existence for just over one year. Which of the following would be the most appropriate action to take to make sure all tasks being performed are included in the new job descriptions?

    a. Ask current staff members to keep a diary for a certain period of time on how they spend their time.

    b. Review job descriptions from other hospitals.

    c. Make random observations of job tasks.

    d. Refer the matter to the human resources department.

117. The scope of performance improvement measurements that help identify important areas of service used by a healthcare organization are:

    a. Structure, process, outcome

    b. Know boundaries, current process, data displays

    c. Risk management, utilization management, safety management

    d. Volume, risk, problem-prone outcomes

Domain VI *Legal*

118. The legal health record:

    a. Is inadmissible into evidence

    b. Will be disclosed upon request

    c. May not be hybrid

    d. Must consist in part on paper

119. Changes to health record entries are:

    a. Acceptable in certain circumstances

    b. Indicative of negligent care

    c. Permissible only in paper health records

    d. Permissible only in electronic health records

120. What is the term used most often to describe the individual within an organization who is responsible for protecting health information in conjunction with the court system?

    a. Administrator of record

    b. Custodian of record

    c. Director of record

    d. Supervisor of record

121. An individual who brings a lawsuit is called the:

    a. Defendant

    b. Plaintiff

    c. Arbitrator

    d. Complainant

122. A hospital health information department receives a subpoena *duces tecum* for records of a former patient. When the health record technician goes to retrieve the patient's medical records, it is discovered that the records being subpoenaed have been purged in accordance with the state retention laws. In this situation, how should the HIM department respond to the subpoena?

    a. Inform defense and plaintiff lawyers that the records no longer exist.

    b. Submit a certification of destruction in response to the subpoena.

    c. Refuse the subpoena since no records exist.

    d. Contact the clerk of the court and explain the situation.

123. Which of the following is a core ethical obligation of HITs?

    a. Coding diseases and operations

    b. Protecting patients' privacy and confidential communications

    c. Transcribing medical reports

    d. Performing quantitative analysis on record content

124. A home health agency plans to implement a computer system whereby its nurses document home care services on a laptop computer taken to the patient's home. The laptops will connect to the agency's computer network. The agency is in the process of identifying strategies to minimize the risks associated with the practice. Which of the following would be the best practice to protect laptop and network data from a virus introduced from an external device?

    a. Session terminations

    b. Encryption

    c. Biometrics

    d. Personal firewall software

125. Community Hospital is implementing a hybrid record. Some documentation will be paper-based and digitally scanned post-discharge. Other parts of the record will be totally electronic. The Medical Record Committee is discussing how interim reports in the health record should be handled. Some on the committee think that all interim reports should be discarded and only the final reports retained in the scanned record. Others take the opposite position. What should the HIM director recommend?

    a. Maintaining only the final results provides the greatest measure of security.

    b. Maintaining only the final results is the best option.

    c. Maintaining all interim reports provides the greatest measure of security.

    d. Maintaining only final reports results in a high volume of duplicate reports.

126. Which of the following ethical principles is being followed when an HIT professional ensures that patient information is only released to those who have a legal right to access it?

    a. Autonomy

    b. Beneficence

    c. Justice

    d. Nonmaleficence

127. A subpoena *duces tecum* compels the recipient to:

    a. Serve on a jury

    b. Answer a complaint

    c. Testify at trial

    d. Bring records to a legal proceeding

128. Which of the following activities is considered an unethical practice?

    a. Backdating progress notes

    b. Performing quantitative analysis

    c. Verifying that an insurance company is one that is authorized to receive patient information

    d. Determining what information is required to fulfill an authorized request for information

129. Physician orders for DNR and DNI should be consistent with:

    a. Patient's advance directive

    b. Patient's bill of rights

    c. Notice of privacy practices

    d. Authorization for release of information

130. When correcting erroneous information in a health record, which of the following is *not* appropriate?

    a. Print "error" above the entry

    b. Enter the correction in chronological sequence

    c. Add the reason for the change

    d. Use black pen to obliterate the entry

131. An individual's right to control access to his or her personal information is known as:

    a. Security

    b. Confidentiality

    c. Privacy

    d. Access control

132. Which of the following ethical principles is being followed when an HIT professional applies rules fairly to all?

    a. Autonomy

    b. Beneficence

    c. Justice

    d. Nonmaleficence

133. A hospital currently includes the patient's social security number on the face sheet of the paper medical record and in the electronic version of the record. The hospital risk manager has identified this as a potential identity fraud risk and wants the information removed. The risk manager is not getting cooperation from the physicians and others in the hospital who say they need the information for identification and other purposes. Given this situation, what should the HIM director suggest?

    a. Avoid displaying the number on any document, screen, or data collection field.

    b. Allow the information in both electronic and paper forms since a variety of people need this data.

    c. Require employees to sign confidentiality agreements if they have access to social security numbers.

    d. Contact legal counsel for advice.

134. Community Hospital is planning implementation of various elements of the EHR in the next six months. Physicians have requested the ability to access the EHR from their offices and from home and to be able to print out the information, if needed. The Medical Record Committee is assessing whether or not to provide this functionality given concerns over patient confidentiality. Given this discussion, what advice should the HIM director provide?

    a. HIPAA regulations do not allow this type of access.

    b. This access would be covered under the release of PHI for treatment purposes and poses no security or confidentiality threats.

    c. Access can be permitted providing that appropriate safeguards are put in place to protect against threats to security.

    d. Access can be permitted because the physicians are on the medical staff of the hospital and are covered by HIPAA as employees.

Revenue Cycle

135. Which of the following actions would be best to determine whether present on admission (POA) indicators for the conditions selected by CMS are having a negative impact on the hospital's Medicare reimbursement?

    a. Identify all records for a period having these indicators for these conditions and determine whether these conditions are the only secondary diagnosis present on the claim that will lead to higher payment.

    b. Identify all records for a period that have these indicators for these conditions.

    c. Identify all records for a period that have these indicators for these conditions and determine whether or not additional documentation can be submitted to Medicare to increase reimbursement.

    d. Take a random sample of records for a period of records having these indicators for these conditions and extrapolate the negative impact on Medicare reimbursement.

136. In processing a bill under the Medicare outpatient prospective payment system (OPPS), in which a patient had three surgical procedures performed during the same operative session, which of the following would apply?

    a. Bundling of services

    b. Outlier adjustment

    c. Pass-through payment

    d. Discounting of procedures

137. Under which prospective payment system are Medicare SNF services paid?

    a. CMGs

    b. DRGs

    c. RBRVS

    d. RUG-III

138. Community Hospital implemented a clinical document improvement (CDI) program six months ago. The goal of the program was to improve clinical documentation to support quality of care, data quality, and HIM coding accuracy. Which of the following would be best to ensure that everyone understands the importance of this program?

    a. Request that the CEO write a memorandum to all hospital staff.

    b. Give the chairperson of the CDI committee authority to fire employees who don't improve their clinical documentation.

    c. Include ancillary clinical and medical staff in the process.

    d. Request a letter from the Joint Commission.

139. The member had had gastric bypass surgery three years previously. As a result of losing over 200 pounds, loose skin hung from the member's arms, thighs, and belly. The member, upon referral from her general surgeon, was scheduled to have a plastic surgeon remove the excess skin. The member called for prior approval as required by the plan. The clinical review resulted in a denial of the surgery as cosmetic. The member requested a peer review and submitted documentation from her physician that the excess skin was causing skin infections and exacerbating her eczema. The peer clinician denied the case. What is the next step in order for the member to have the surgery paid for by her insurance company?

a. File a lawsuit

b. Appeal to an expert clinician in the same specialty

c. Schedule the surgery with her original general surgeon as that surgeon was paid

d. Disenroll from the plan and enroll with indemnity healthcare insurance

140. A pharmacist who submits Medicaid claims for reimbursement on brand name drugs when less expensive generic drugs were actually dispensed has committed the crime of:

a. Criminal negligence

b. Fraud

c. Perjury

d. Products' liability

141. Which of the following departments are responsible for revenue cycle management in a hospital?

a. Volunteer services, admitting, and housekeeping

b. Patient financial services, health information management, and admitting

c. Admitting, food services, and accounting

d. Health information management, billing, and volunteer services

142. The process of attaching an HCPCS code to a procedure so that the code will automatically be included on the patient's bill is known by which of the following terms?

a. Chargemaster

b. Hard coding

c. Price compendium

d. Insurance code mapping

143. In a typical acute-care setting, Admitting is located in which revenue cycle area?

a. Pre-claims submission

b. Claims processing

c. Accounts receivable

d. Claims reconciliation/collections

144. The concept of the revenue cycle originated out of the healthcare facility's need to structure services to meet the changing and challenging demands for:

    a. Increasing accuracy required of outpatient coding

    b. Reducing the number of accounts on the "discharged, not final billed" report

    c. Reimbursement from third-party payers, compliance, and demands for greater efficiencies to enhance revenue

    d. Better information to be collected and processed by registration and patient accounting departments

145. Accounts receivable (AR) refers to charges for patient services that are:

    a. Waiting to be billed to the insurance company or third-party payer

    b. Only in-house hospital charges that have been billed

    c. Only discharged patient charges that are unbilled

    d. Already billed to insurance companies and are awaiting payment

146. The phrase "aging of accounts" refers to accounts that have been:

    a. Billed but not paid

    b. Discharged but not billed

    c. Admitted but not discharged

    d. Paid but not credited

147. In preparing a bill for Mr. Smith's healthcare services, the health record technician needs to determine those services to be paid under Medicare Part A and those under Medicare Part B. Which of the following services should be processed under Part B?

    a. Inpatient hospitalization care

    b. Inpatient laboratory and radiology services

    c. Skilled nursing facility care

    d. Surgeon's services

148. Which of the following coding error classifications is most valuable in determining the impact on overall revenue cycle?

    a. Errors by coding guideline

    b. Percentage of cases that could have been improved if queried

    c. Errors by coder

    d. Errors that produced changes in MS-DRG assignment

149. An HIM director is requesting the purchase of a document imaging system. However, the Hospital Budget Committee is reluctant to approve the request because of the expense. The committee thinks that the money is better spent implementing CPOE and other EHR applications. Which of the following might the HIM director use as a cost–benefit justification?

    a. The EHR system will take too long to implement.

    b. The Joint Commission requires that the hospital move to digital scanning.

    c. "Discharged, not final billed" and accounts receivable days can be improved because of workflow efficiencies.

    d. HIPAA requires the use of digital tracking of release of information.

150. The Patient Accounting department at Wildcat Hospital is concerned because last night's bill drop contained half the usual number of inpatient cases. Which of the following reports will be most useful in determining the reason for the low volume of bills?

a. Accounts Receivable Aging Report

b. Accounts Not Selected for Billing Report

c. Case-Mix Index Report

d. Discharge Summary Report

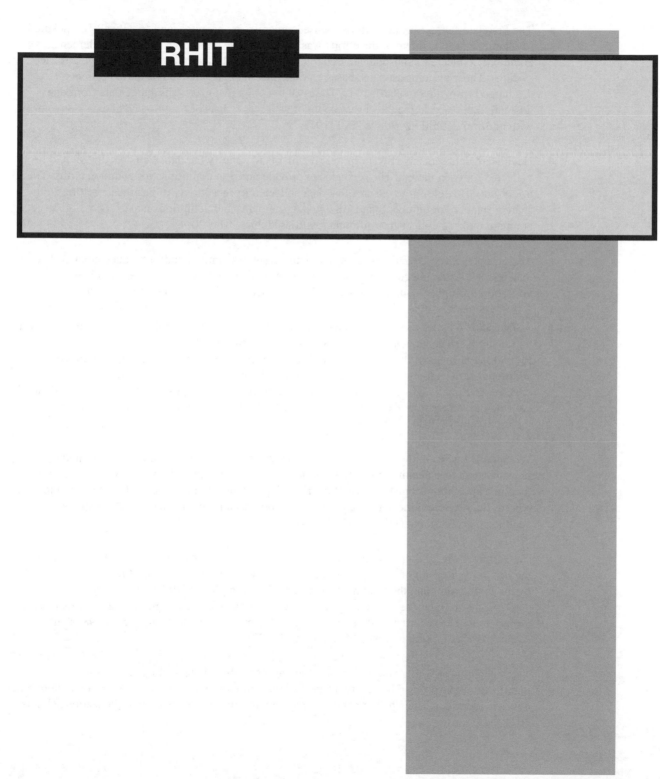

RHIT

Answer
Key

Practice Answers

1. **d** In many facilities, the director of health information services leads the system's clinical data standards committee. A critical early step in implementing the EHR is to develop a data dictionary (Johns 2011, 199).

2. **a** The first data standardization efforts focused generally on hospitals and specifically on hospital discharge data. The intent of the efforts was to standardize definitions of key data elements commonly collected in hospitals. Discharge data were collected in hospital discharge abstract systems. These systems used databases compiled from aggregate data on all the patients discharged from a particular facility. The need to compare uniform discharge data from one hospital to the next led to the development of data sets or lists of recommended data elements with uniform definitions (Johns 2011, 197).

3. **a** Healthcare data sets have two purposes: the first is to identify the data elements that should be collected for each patient. The second is to provide uniform definitions for common terms. The use of uniform definitions ensures that data collected from a variety of healthcare settings will share a standard definition. Standardizing data elements and definitions makes it possible to compare the data collected at different facilities (Johns 2011, 201).

★ 4. **a** The purpose of the UHDDS is to list and define a set of common, uniform data elements. The data elements are collected from the health records of every hospital inpatient and later abstracted from the health record and included in national databases (Johns 2011, 202).

5. **b** A data set is a list of recommended data elements with uniform definitions that are relevant for a particular use. The contents of data sets vary by their purpose. However, data sets are not meant to limit the number of data elements that can be collected. Most healthcare organizations collect additional data elements that have meaning for their specific administrative and clinical operations. Standardizing data elements and definitions makes it possible to compare the data collected at different facilities. A number of data reporting requirements come from federal initiatives (Johns 2011, 202–203).

6. **a** When deficiencies in the health record, such as reports that need to be dictated or signed by a physician or other health professional, are identified through quantitative analysis, the record is filed in a specially designated area of the HIM department, frequently called the incomplete record file. A copy of the deficiency slip also is filed, usually by the name of the responsible healthcare professional (Johns 2011, 411–412).

7. **b** The terminal-digit filing system is considered by many to be the most efficient. In this system, the last digit or group of last digits (terminal digits) is the primary unit used for filing, followed by the middle unit and the last unit of numbers. For example, 443798 could be broken down as 44-37-98, with 98 as the primary unit for filing, 37 as the secondary (middle) unit, and 44 as the tertiary unit. The record would be filed in the following arrangement: file section, 98; shelf number, 37; and folder number, 44 (Johns 2011, 393).

★ 8. **a** The alphanumeric filing system uses a combination of alpha letters and numbers for identification purposes. The first two letters of the patient's last name are followed by a unique numeric identifier. The alphanumeric filing system is appropriate for small organizations (Johns 2011, 382).

9. **d** Timeliness of the storage and retrieval processes can be monitored. In this situation each clinic visit represents a patient record that will need to be retrieved (or pulled) and stored (filed back), 600 / 60 = 10; 600 / 40 = 15; 10 + 15 = 25 hours per day (Johns 2011, 418).

10. **b** In the unit numbering system, the patient receives a unique health record number at the time of the first encounter. For all subsequent encounters for a particular patient, the health record number that was assigned for the first encounter is used (Johns 2011, 388).

11. **b** In alphabetical filing systems, records are arranged in alphabetical order. This system is usually satisfactory for a very small volume of records, such as records maintained in small physician practices. For organizations that have thousands of records, however, alphabetical filing has many disadvantages. First, it does not ensure a unique identifier. A second disadvantage is that alphabetical files do not expand evenly. Statistically, almost half the files fall under the letters *B, C, H, M, S,* and *W.* A third disadvantage to the alphabetical filing system is that it is time-consuming to purge or clean out files for inactive storage. With an alphabetical filing system, each individual record needs to be checked for the last patient encounter to determine whether it is inactive (Johns 2011, 391).

12. **b** A requisition is a request from a clinical or other area in the organization to charge out a specific health record. The requisition may be in paper or electronic form. The information contained on a requisition usually includes patient's name, health record number, date of the request, date and time needed, name of the requestor, and location for delivery (Johns 2011, 403).

13. **b** Some small facilities and clinics use an alphabetical patient identification and filing system. In this system, the patient's last name is used as the first source of identification and his or her first name and middle initial provide further identification. The disadvantage to this system is that a given community may have several persons with the same or a similar name. In this case, the facility routinely uses date of birth as the next step in the process of identifying a patient (Johns 2011, 392).

14. **d** Some case-mix systems use the CMI as a basis for reimbursement. In that way, the CMI also is a measure of the average revenue received per case. Many hospitals closely monitor the movement of their CMI for inpatient populations for which payment is based on DRGs and for outpatient populations for which payment is based on APCs (Schraffenberger and Kuehn 2011, 483).

15. **c** Tracking the location of health records removed from a paper-based storage system area is key to ensuring their accessibility to authorized persons. The outguide is the most common type of tracking system used to track paper-based health records. An outguide is usually made of strong colored vinyl with two plastic pockets. It is the size of a regular record folder and is placed in the record location when the record is removed from the file (Johns 2011, 402).

16. **b** The goals of the HIPAA security rule are to ensure the confidentiality, integrity, and availability of the ePHI. Integrity is ensuring that data are not altered either during transmission across a network or during storage. ePHI must be available when needed for patient care and other uses (Sayles and Trawick 2010, 300).

17. **d** The terminal-digit filing system is considered by many to be the most efficient. In this system, the last digit or group of last digits (terminal digits) is the primary unit used for filing, followed by the middle unit and the last unit of numbers. For example, 443798 could be broken down as 44-37-98, with 98 as the primary unit for filing, 37 as the secondary (middle) unit, and 44 as the tertiary unit. The record would be filed in the following arrangement: file section, 98; shelf number, 37; and folder number, 44 (Johns 2011, 393).

18. **a** In 1969, a conference on hospital discharge abstract systems was sponsored jointly by NCHS, the National Center for Health Services Research and Development, and Johns Hopkins University. Conference participants recommended that all short-term general hospitals in the United States collect a minimum set of patient-specific data elements. They also recommended that these data elements be included in all databases compiled from hospital discharge abstract systems (Johns 2011, 202).

✱ 19. **c** The data collected by the MDS are used to develop a resident assessment protocol (RAP) summary for each resident. The MDS provides a structured way to organize resident information and develop a resident care plan. Problems identified through the assessment process are documented and a RAP is triggered (Johns 2011, 208).

20. **a** Workflow support also has been added to EDMSs. This means that the EDMS facilitates various functions that must be performed, often simultaneously or in a specific sequence (Johns 2011, 143, 164).

✱ 21. **a** Data granularity requires that the attributes and values of data be defined at the correct level of detail for the intended use of the data (Johns 2011, 48).

✱ 22. **b** To support the development of networked health information systems, NHIN defines three dimensions of the infrastructure that provide a means for conceptualizing the capture, storage, communication, processing, and presentation of information for each group of information users. A set of core data elements has been developed for each dimension as part of the NCVHS report (Johns 2011, 213).

23. **a** The continuity of care record (CCR) standard (ASTM E2369-05) is a core data set of relevant administrative, demographic, and clinical information elements about a patient's health status and healthcare treatment (ASTM 2009). It was created to help communicate that information from one provider to another for referral, transfer, or discharge of the patient (Johns 2011, 226).

24. **b** The Outcomes and Assessment Information Set (OASIS-C) is a standardized data set designed to gather data about Medicare beneficiaries who are receiving services from a home health agency. OASIS-C includes a set of core data items that are collected on all adult home health patients (Johns 2011, 209).

25. **d** The Health Plan Employer Data and Information Set (HEDIS) is sponsored by the National Committee for Quality Assurance (NCQA). HEDIS is a set of standard performance measures designed to provide healthcare purchasers and consumers with the information they need to compare the performance of managed healthcare plans (Johns 2011, 210).

26. **d** The purpose of a database is to store and retrieve data. A popular common language called structured query language (SQL) is used to store and retrieve data in relational databases. SQL gives the information system the ability to query and report on data and to insert, update, and delete data from the database (Johns 2011, 903–904).

27. **c**   The MPI functions as the primary guide to locating pertinent demographic data about the patient and his or her health record number. Without the information contained in the MPI, it would be almost impossible to locate a patient's health record in most organizations that use a numeric filing system. The MPI is the permanent record of every patient ever seen in the healthcare entity. The amount of information contained on each patient in the MPI varies from facility to facility. However, the basic information usually includes: patient's last, first, and middle names; patient's health record number(s); Patient's date of birth; Patient's gender; dates of encounter. Additional information such as address, telephone number, and attending physician for each encounter also may be recorded in the index (Johns 2011, 484).

28. **a**   Some providers also use a SOAP format for their problem-oriented progress notes. A subjective (S) entry relates significant information in the patient's words or from the patient's point of view (Johns 2011, 114).

29. **c**   Some providers also use a SOAP format for their problem-oriented progress notes. Professional conclusions reached from evaluation of the subjective or objective information make up the assessment (A) (Johns 2011, 114).

30. **d**   Standardized vocabulary is needed to facilitate the indexing, storage, and retrieval of patient information in an EHR. SNOMED CT creates a standardized vocabulary. The Computer-based Patient Record Institute (CPRI) has studied the ability of current nomenclatures to capture information for EHRs. The institute has determined that SNOMED CT is the most comprehensive controlled vocabulary for coding the contents of the health record and facilitating the development of computerized records (Johns 2011, 260–261).

31. **d**   *International Classification of Diseases, Ninth Revision, Clinical Modification* (ICD-9-CM), including the Official ICD-9-CM Guidelines for Coding and Reporting: Volumes 1 and 2 are used for reporting all diseases, injuries, impairments, other health problems and causes of such, and Volume 3 is used to report procedures performed on hospital inpatients (Johns 2011, 238).

32. **a**   Although sometimes used interchangeably, the terms *data* and *information* do not mean the same thing. Data represent the basic facts about people, processes, measurements, conditions, and so on. They can be collected in the form of dates, numerical measurements and statistics, textual descriptions, checklists, images, and symbols. After data have been collected and analyzed, they are converted into a form that can be used for a specific purpose. This useful form is called information. In other words, data represent facts and information represents meaning (Johns 2011, 28–29).

33. **b**   Structure and content standards establish and provide clear and uniform definitions of the data elements to be included in EHR systems. They specify the type of data to be collected in each data field and the attributes and values of each data field, all of which are captured in data dictionaries (Johns 2011, 225).

34. **c**   The terminal-digit filing system is considered by many to be the most efficient. In this system, the last digit or group of last digits (terminal digits) is the primary unit used for filing, followed by the middle unit and the last unit of numbers. For example, 443798 could be broken down as 44-37-98, with 98 as the primary unit for filing, 37 as the secondary (middle) unit, and 44 as the tertiary unit. The record would be filed in the following arrangement: file section, 98; shelf number, 37; and folder number, 44 (Johns 2011, 393).

35. **c** Data currency and data timeliness mean that healthcare data should be up-to-date and recorded at or near the time of the event or observation. Because care and treatment rely on accurate and current data, an essential characteristic of data quality is the timeliness of the documentation or data entry (Johns 2011, 48).

36. **b** Data consistency means that the data are reliable. Reliable data do not change no matter how many times or in how many ways they are stored, processed, or displayed. Data values are consistent when the value of any given data element is the same across applications and systems. Related data items also should be reliable (Johns 2011, 47).

37. **d** Scatter diagrams are used to plot the points for two continuous variables that may be related to each other in some way. For example, one might want to look at whether age and blood pressure are related. One variable, age, would be plotted on the vertical axis of the graph, and the other variable, blood pressure, would be plotted on the horizontal axis (Johns 2011, 632).

38. **d** Both *x* and *y* axes are in unequal measures, so data are not accurately represented. Line graphs are used to display time trends as opposed to a histogram or bar chart (Johns 2011, 540).

39. **a** Efficiency is another component of health record storage that will be improved in computer-based systems. Providing access to paper-based health records is an inefficient process, especially when information must be transferred between providers and facilities. Even internal transfers of health records can be troublesome because paper records may be needed in more than one place at a time. Moreover, paper records can be easily misplaced by users or misfiled by staff (Johns 2011, 50).

40. **c** Besides storage of patient care documentation, the health record has other equally important functions. These include helping physicians, nurses, and other caregivers make diagnoses and choose treatment options. Invoices for services would not be part of the physician record (Johns 2011, 42).

41. **d** The data quality model applies the following quality characteristics: data accuracy, data accessibility, data comprehensiveness, data consistency, data currency, data definition, data granularity, data precision, data relevancy, and data timeliness (Johns 2011, 43–44).

42. **b** Line graphs are used to display time trends in data. A line graph is useful for plotting data to make observations. In analyzing the chart, the revenue exceeds the costs (Johns, 2011, 540–542).

43. **c** Data granularity requires that the attributes and values of data be defined at the correct level of detail for the intended use of the data. For example, numerical values for laboratory results should be recorded to the appropriate decimal place as required for the meaningful interpretation of test results—or in the collection of demographic data, data elements should be defined appropriately to determine the differences in outcomes of care among various populations (Johns 2011, 48).

44. **a** Patient care delivery is a primary purpose of the health record. Other primary purposes are patient care management, patient care support processes, financial and other administrative processes, and patient self-management (Johns 2011, 30–31).

45. **c** Data comprehensiveness means that all the required data elements are included in the health record. In essence, comprehensiveness means that the record is complete. In both paper-based and computer-based systems, having a complete health record is critical to the organization's ability to provide excellent patient care and to meet all regulatory, legal, and reimbursement requirements (Johns 2011, 46).

46. **b** Data accessibility means that the data are easily obtainable. Any organization that maintains health records for individual patients must have systems in place that identify each patient and support efficient access to information on each patient. Authorized users of the health record must be able to access information easily when and where they need it (Johns 2011, 46).

47. **b** The health record number (also called the medical record number) is a key data element in the MPI. It is used as a unique personal identifier and is also used in paper-based numerical filing systems to locate records and in electronic systems to link records. Although it is typically assigned at the point of patient registration, the HIM department is usually responsible for the integrity of health record number assignment and for ensuring that no two patients receive the same number (Johns 2011, 386–387).

48. **c** The operative report describes the surgical procedures performed on the patient. The operative report should be written or dictated by the surgeon immediately after surgery and become part of the health record (Johns 2011, 71, 73).

49. **a** The results of all diagnostic and therapeutic procedures become part of the patient's health record. The medical laboratory report includes tests performed on blood, urine, and other samples from the patient (Johns 2011, 70).

50. **b** The discharge summary is a concise account of the patient's illness, course of treatment, response to treatment, and condition at the time the patient is discharged (officially released) from the hospital. The summary also includes instructions for follow-up care to be given to the patient or his or her caregiver at the time of discharge. It provides an overview of the entire medical encounter. The discharge summary is the responsibility of, and must be signed by, the attending physician (Johns 2011, 78).

51. **b** Nurses maintain chronological records of the patient's vital signs (blood pressure, heart rate, respiration rate, and temperature) and separate logs that show what medications were ordered and when they were administered (Johns 2011, 68).

52. **a** The health record generally contains two types of data: clinical and administrative. Clinical data document the patient's medical condition, diagnosis, and procedures performed as well as the healthcare treatment provided. Administrative data include demographic and financial information as well as various consents and authorizations related to the provision of care and the handling of confidential patient information (Johns 2011, 61).

53. **c** Information usually documented in the physical examination includes vital signs and head, eyes, ears, nose, throat (HEENT) (Johns 2011, 63, 65).

54. **d** Digital scanners create images of handwritten and printed documents that are then store in health record databases as electronic files. The data can be interfaced in the current EHR with the document scanning system. Using scanned images solves many of the problems associated with traditional paper-based health records and hybrid records (Odom-Wesley et al. 2009, 227).

55. **c**   Documentation of these results would typically be found in the ECG report (Johns 2011, 70–71).

56. **d**   This documentation would typically be found in social service notes (Johns 2011, 68).

57. **c**   Information typically included in the patient's health record for an emergency visit includes: patient's instructions at discharge, time and means of patient's arrival, emergency care administered before arrival at the facility, clinical observations, etc. The patient's complete medical history would not be included in the record (Johns 2011, 93).

✗ 58. **b**   The problem-oriented health record is better suited to serve the patient and the end user of the patient information. The key characteristic of this format is an itemized list of the patient's past and present social, psychological, and medical problems. Each problem is indexed with a unique number (Johns 2011, 114).

59. **d**   The third major type of paper-based health record is the integrated health record. The integrated health record is arranged so that the documentation from various sources is intermingled and follows strict chronological order. The advantage of the integrated format is that it is easy to follow the course of the patient's diagnosis and treatment. The disadvantage is that the format makes it difficult to compare similar types of information (Johns 2011, 114).

60. **b**   A complete medical history documents the patient's current complaints and symptoms and lists his or her past medical, personal, and family history. In acute care, the medical history is usually the responsibility of the attending physician (Johns 2011, 62–63).

61. **a**   The physical examination report represents the attending physician's assessment of the patient's current health status. This report should document information on all the patient's major organ systems (Johns 2011, 63, 65).

✗ 62. **b**   The consultation report documents the clinical opinion of a physician other than the primary or attending physician. The consultation is requested by the primary or attending physician. The report is based on the consulting physician's examination of the patient and a review of his or her health record (Johns 2011, 78).

✗ 63. **c**   The secondary purposes of the health record are not associated with specific encounters between patient and healthcare professional. Rather, they are related to the environment in which patient care is provided. Some secondary purposes are: support for research, to serve as evidence in litigation, to allocate resources, to plan market strategy, etc. (Johns 2011, 31–32).

64. **a**   Patient care management refers to all the activities related to managing the healthcare services provided to patients and is a primary purpose of the health record. The health record assists providers in analyzing various illnesses, formulating practice guidelines, and evaluating the quality of care (Johns 2011, 31).

✗ 65. **b**   The American Society for Testing and Materials (ASTM) is an SDO that develops standards for a variety of industries in the United States. The ASTM Technical Committee on Healthcare Informatics E31 is charged with the responsibility for developing standards related to the EHR. E31 works through subcommittees assigned to various aspects of this endeavor. The continuity of care record (CCR) standard (ASTM E2369-05) is a core data set of relevant administrative, demographic, and clinical information elements about a patient's health status and healthcare treatment (ASTM 2009). It was created to help communicate that information from one provider to another for referral, transfer, or discharge of the patient (Johns 2011, 225–226).

66. **a** HL7 is a standards development organization accredited by the American National Standards Institute that addresses issues at the seventh, or application, level of healthcare systems interconnections. It develops messaging, data content, and document standards to support the exchange of clinical information (Johns 2011, 224).

67. **b** Digital scanners create images of handwritten and printed documents that are then store in health record databases as electronic files. The data can be interfaced in the current EHR with the document scanning system. Performing the scanning function concurrently improves the ability for the HIM staff to ensure completeness of the health record (Odom-Wesley et al. 2009, 227).

68. **b** The term *information* refers to data that have been collected, combined, analyzed, interpreted, and/or converted into a form that can be used for specific purposes. In other words, data represent facts; information represents meaning (Johns 2011, 197).

69. **c** Consistency is sometimes referred to as data *reliability*. For example, all patients in a trauma registry with the same level, severity, and site of injury should have the same score on the Abbreviated Injury Scale. Reliability is frequently checked by having more than one person abstract data for the same case. The results are then compared to identify any discrepancies (Johns 2011, 509).

70. **c** Mortality is a term referring to the incidence of death in a specific population or the loss of subjects during the course of a clinical research study (Johns 2011, 247, 523).

71. **b** Cancer registries were developed as an organized method to collect these data. Case finding is a method used to identify the patients who have been seen and/or treated in the facility for the particular disease or condition of interest to the registry. After cases have been identified, extensive information is abstracted from the patients' paper-based health records into the registry database or extracted from other databases and automatically entered into the registry database (Johns 2011, 485–486, 509).

72. **d** Several organizations have developed standards or approval processes for cancer programs. The American College of Surgeons (ACS) Commission on Cancer has an approval process for cancer programs. One of the requirements of this process is the existence of a cancer registry as part of the program (Johns 2011, 488).

73. **b** Data for the National Survey of Ambulatory Surgery are collected on a representative sample of hospital-based and freestanding ambulatory surgery centers. Data include patient demographic characteristics, source of payment; information on anesthesia given, the diagnoses, and the surgical and nonsurgical procedures on patient visits of hospital-based and freestanding ambulatory surgery centers (Johns 2011, 500).

74. **c** The disease index is a listing in diagnosis code number order for patients discharged from the facility during a particular time period. Each patient's diagnoses are converted from a verbal description to a numerical code, usually using the *International Classification of Diseases*. The patient's diagnosis codes are entered into the facility's health information system as part of the discharge processing of the patient's health record (Johns 2011, 485).

75. **d** The Operation Index is similar to the Disease Index except that it is arranged in numerical order by the patient's procedure code(s) using International Classification of Diseases or *Current Procedural Terminology* (CPT) codes (Johns 2011, 484–485).

✸ 76. **a**   Case finding is a method used to identify the patients who have been seen and/or treated in the facility for the particular disease or condition of interest to the registry. After cases have been identified, extensive information is abstracted from the patients' paper-based health records into the registry database or extracted from other databases and automatically entered into the registry database (Johns 2011, 485–486).

✸ 77. **b**   When a case is first entered in the registry, an accession number is assigned. This number consists of the first digits of the year the patient was first seen at the facility, and the remaining digits are assigned sequentially throughout the year. The first case in the year, for example, might be 10-0001. The accession number may be assigned manually or by the automated cancer database used by the organization (Johns 2011, 487).

78. **b**   Vital statistics include data on births, deaths, fetal deaths, marriages, and divorces. Responsibility for the collection of vital statistics rests with the states (Johns 2011, 501–502).

✸ 79. **c**   Although registries and databases are almost universally computerized, data collection is commonly done manually, not all data collection is done manually. In some cases, data can be downloaded directly from other electronic systems. Birth defect registries, for example, often download information on births and birth defects from the vital records system. In some cases, providers such as hospitals and physicians send information in electronic format to the registry or database. As the electronic health record (EHR) develops further, less and less data will need to be manually abstracted since it will be available electronically through the EHR (Johns 2011, 507).

80. **a**   The health record is considered a primary data source because it contains information about a patient that has been documented by the professionals who provided care or services to that patient. Data taken from the primary health record and entered into registries and databases are considered a secondary data source (Johns 2011, 481).

81. **a**   Secondary data are considered aggregate data. Aggregate data include data on groups of people or patients without identifying any particular patient individually. Examples of aggregate data are statistics on the average length of stay (ALOS) for patients discharged within a particular diagnosis-related group (DRG) (Johns 2011, 481–482).

82. **c**   A proportion is a type of ratio in which x is a portion of the whole ($x + y$). In a proportion, the numerator is always included in the denominator (Johns 2011, 525).

✸ 83. **b**   The range is the simplest measure of spread. It is the difference between the smallest and largest values in a frequency distribution (Johns 2011, 532–533).

84. **c**   The mean is the arithmetic average of frequency distribution. Put simply, it is the sum of all the values in a frequency distribution divided by the frequency: $(10 + 15 + 20 + 25 + 25) / 5 = 19$ (Johns 2011, 529).

85. **a**   The average length of stay (ALOS) is calculated from the total LOS. The total LOS divided by the number of patients discharged is the average length of stay (ALOS) (Johns 2011, 553).

86. **c**   A *hospital inpatient is a* person who is provided room, board, and continuous general nursing service in an area of the hospital where patients generally stay at least overnight. A *hospital outpatient is a* hospital patient who receives services in one or more of the outpatient facilities when not currently an inpatient or home care patient (Johns 2011, 546–547).

87. **a**   The mode is the simplest measure of central tendency. It is used to indicate the most frequent observation is a frequency distribution. The most frequent observation is 30 (Johns 2011, 531–532).

88. **c**   A table should contain all the information the user needs to understand the data in it. One of the things it should have is no blank cells. When no information is available for a particular cell, the cell should contain a zero (Johns 2011, 535).

89. **c**   Length of stay (LOS) is calculated for each patient after he/she is discharged from the hospital. It is the number of calendar days from the day of patient admission to the day of discharge $(31 - 21) + 1 = 11$ days (Johns 2011, 553).

90. **c**   The median is the midpoint of a frequency distribution. It is the point at which 50% of observations fall above and 50% fall below. Eight is the mid-point of the distribution where 50% of the observations fall above and below 8 (Johns 2011, 531).

91. **c**   The gross autopsy rate is the proportion or percentage of deaths that are followed by the performance of autopsy. $(5 / 25) \times 100 = 20\%$ (Johns 2011, 561).

92. **d**   A pie chart is an easily understood chart in which the sizes of the slices of the pie show the proportional contribution of each part. Pie charts can be used to show the component parts of a single group or variable (Johns 2011, 537).

93. **b**   An incidence rate is used to compare the frequency of disease in different populations. Populations are compared using rates instead of raw numbers because rates adjust for differences in population size. The incidence rate is the probability or risk of illness in a population over a period of time (Johns 2011, 576).

94. **d**   The result of the official count taken at midnight is the daily inpatient census. This is the number of inpatients present at the official census-taking time each day. Also included in the daily inpatient census are any patients who were admitted and discharged the same day (Johns 2011, 547).

95. **a**   A unit of measure that reflects the services received by one inpatient during a 24-hour period is an inpatient service day (IPSD). The number of inpatient service days for a 24-hour period is equal to the daily inpatient census, that is, one service day for each patient treated (Johns 2011, 548).

96. **c**   The gross hospital death rate is the proportion of all hospital discharges that ended in death. It is the basic indicator of mortality in a healthcare facility. The gross death rate is calculated by dividing the total number of deaths occurring in a given time period by the total number of discharges, including deaths, for the same time period (Johns 2011, 556).

97. **b**   Length of stay (LOS) is calculated for each patient after he or she is discharged from the hospital. It is the number of calendar days from the day of patient admission to the day of discharge. When the patient is admitted and discharged in the same month, the LOS is determined by subtracting the date of admission from the date of discharge (Johns 2011, 553).

98. **b**   A gross autopsy rate is the proportion or percentage of deaths that are followed by the performance of autopsy (Johns 2011, 561).

99. **b** Even though much of the data collection process has been automated, an ongoing responsibility of the HIM professional is to verify the census data that are collected daily. The census reports patient activity for a 24-hour reporting period. Included in the census report are the number of inpatients admitted and discharged for the previous 24-hour period and the number of intrahospital transfers. An intrahospital transfer is a patient who is moved from one patient care unit (for example, the intensive care unit) to another (for example, the surgical unit). The usual 24-hour reporting period begins at 12:01 a.m. and ends at 12:00 p.m. (midnight). In the census count, adults and children are reported separately from newborns (Johns 2011, 547).

100. **c** The result of the official count taken at midnight is the daily inpatient census (Johns 2011, 547).

101. **a** OBRA required CMS to develop an assessment instrument to standardize the collection of SNF patient data. That instrument is known as the resident assessment instrument (RAI) and includes the Minimum Data Set 3.0 (MDS) (Johns 2011, 328).

102. **c** Internal users of patient data are individuals located within the healthcare facility. Examples of internal users are medical staff and administrative and management staff. The hospital administrator would be an internal user of patient information, and the other three choices are all external to the healthcare organization and would be external users of data (Johns 2011, 483).

103. **a** A clinical trial is a research project in which new treatments and tests are investigated to determine whether they are safe and effective. The trial proceeds according to a protocol, which is the list of rules and procedures to be followed. Clinical trials databases have been developed to allow physicians and patients to find clinical trials (Johns 2011, 502–503).

104. **c** Under the IRF-PPS system, each patient is assigned to a case-mix group (CMG) and a tier within the CMG. The CMG assignment is based on the primary condition for which the patient was admitted to the IRF or inpatient unit and on the patient's functional and cognitive abilities at the time of the admission. The tier assignment is based on the presence of one or more specified secondary diagnoses, or comorbidities, that affect the resources needed to treat the patient. Each CMG and tier is assigned a relative weight (RW) that serves as the basis for the payment rate. The payment rate is adjusted at the facility level for teaching status, the applicable geographic wage index, and the percentage of low-income patients served by the facility. Cases with extraordinary high costs compared to the prospectively set payment may qualify for an outlier payment (Schraffenberger and Kuehn 2011, 480–481).

105. **d** A fourth digit code must be used when present. Diagnosis is of eyelid, 216.1, is correct code (Schraffenberger 2012, 29).

106. **b** The excludes notes found in the Tabular List are hard to miss because the word *excludes* appears in italicized print with a box around it. The exclusion note indicates that code 210.0, rather than code 216.0, should be assigned if the skin of the lip is the vermilion border of the lip (Schraffenberger 2012, 18).

107. **d** During surgery, physicians may take some normal-looking skin around the growth. Removal of the normal-looking skin is known as taking margins. This is done to be sure no cancer cells are left behind. The total size of the excised area, including margins, is needed for accurate coding. Usually, this information is provided in the operative report (Smith 2012, 59–60).

108. **a** A complex repair of a wound goes beyond layer closure and requires scar revision, debridement, extensive undermining, stents, or retention sutures (Smith 2012, 65).

109. **d**   Signs and symptoms integral to the disease process should not be coded. In this case the nausea, vomiting, and abdominal pain are integral to the acute cholecystitis (Schraffenberger 2012, Appendix I, 11).

110. **a**   This patient's sepsis has resolved before being admitted to the hospital and would be considered a previous condition. She is treated with an aspiration dilation and curettage with products of conception found. The patient's principal diagnosis would be the miscarriage (Schraffenberger 2012, 71).

111. **c**   As a result of the disparity in documentation practices by providers, querying has become a common communication and educational method to advocate proper documentation practices. Queries can be made in situations when there is clinical evidence for a higher degree of specificity or severity (Schraffenberger and Kuehn 2011, 42).

112. **b**   Upcoding is the practice of using a code that results in a higher payment to the provider that actually reflects the service of item provided (Schraffenberger and Kuehn 2011, 372).

113. **c**   The principal diagnosis is designated and defined as the condition established after study to chiefly responsible for occasioning the admission of the patient to the hospital for care (Schraffenberger 2012, 68).

114. **b**   The principal diagnosis is designated and defined as the condition established after study to chiefly responsible for occasioning the admission of the patient to the hospital for care. The abdominal pain would not be coded as it is a symptom of the gastroenteritis (Schraffenberger 2012, 68).

115. **c**   A patient may have a history of a primary site of malignancy but later develop a secondary neoplasm or a metastatic site at another location. When this occurs, the treatment is likely to be directed to the secondary site. The secondary site code (196–199) is assigned first with a category V10 codes used as an additional diagnosis code (Schraffenberger 2012, 110–111).

116. **a**   Two or more diagnoses that equally meet the definition for principal diagnosis: In the unusual instance when two or more diagnoses equally meet the criteria for principal diagnosis, as determined by the circumstances of admission, diagnostic workup, and/or the therapy provided, and the Alphabetic Index, Tabular List, or another coding guideline does not provide sequencing in such cases, any one of the diagnoses may be sequenced first (Schraffenberger 2012, 68–69).

117. **c**   Other diagnoses are designated and defined as all conditions that coexist at the time of admission, that develop subsequently, or that affect the treatment received and/or the length of stay (LOS). Diagnoses are to be excluded that related to an earlier episode that has no bearing on the current hospital stay (Schraffenberger 2012, 71).

118. **c**   The patient has the signs and symptoms and responded to treatment that would be given because of asthma with status asthmaticus. The physician can be queried based on the clinical indicators of a diagnosis when no documentation of the condition is present (Schraffenberger and Kuehn 2011, 42).

119. **b**   Procardia is an antianginal, antihypertensive, calcium channel blocker that is used to treat stable angina pectoris, vasospastic angina, and hypertension (Schraffenberger 2012, Appendix D, 14).

120. **b** Signs, symptoms, abnormal test results, or other reasons for the outpatient visit are used when a physician qualifies a diagnostic statement as "possible," "probable," "suspected," "questionable," "rule out," or "working diagnosis," or other similar terms indicating uncertainty (Schraffenberger 2012, 343–344).

121. **d** Code T for APC 0044 designates that the APC payment is subject to payment reduction when multiple procedures are performed during the same visit. In the case, there were no additional procedures so the status indicator does not affect payment (Smith 2012, 259).

122. **b** HCPCS (pronounced *hick picks*) is a collection of codes and descriptors used to represent healthcare procedures, supplies, products, and services (Johns 2011, 253).

123. **c** *The International Classification of Diseases for Oncology,* Third Edition (ICD-O-3) is a system used for classifying incidences of malignant disease. Hospitals use ICD-O-3 for several purposes, for example, to develop cancer registries. Cancer registries list all the cases of cancer diagnosed and treated in the facility (Johns 2011, 251).

124. **b** Septicemia generally refers to a systemic disease associated with the presence of pathological microorganisms or toxins in the blood, which can include bacteria, viruses, fungi, or other organisms. Code 038.11 is for septicemia with *Staphylococcus aureus*. Because abdominal pain is a symptom of diverticulitis, only the diverticulitis of the colon is coded (Schraffenberger 2012, 80–81).

125. **d** In the field of medicine, two physicians may use two different terms for the same medical condition. This makes it difficult to gather and retrieve information. Standardized vocabulary is needed to facilitate the indexing, storage, and retrieval of patient information in an EHR. SNOMED CT creates a standardized vocabulary (Johns 2011, 259–260).

126. **d** To assign these codes, documentation in the health record must support a causal relationship. When a causal relationship exists, the principal diagnosis code assigned is a diabetic code from category 250, followed by the code for the manifestation or complication. The diabetes codes and the secondary codes that correspond to them are paired codes that follow the etiology/manifestation convention of the classification. With no documentation as to the type of diabetes, the default is Type 2, with the fifth digit of 0 (Schraffenberger 2012, 124)

127. **d** Volumes 1 and 2 of the *International Classification of Diseases, Ninth Revision, Clinical Modification* (ICD-9-CM), including the Official ICD-9-CM Guidelines for Coding and Reporting: Volumes 1 and 2, are used for reporting all diseases, injuries, impairments, other health problems and causes of such. ICD-9-CM Volumes 1 and 2 will be replaced with ICD-10-CM (Johns 2011, 238).

128. **d** ICD-9-CM is the most recognized classification system used today in the United States. It evolved from a classification developed by Dr. Jacques Bertillon. This classification system was revised throughout the early 1900s. In 1948, the World Health Organization (WHO) published the Sixth Revision of the system. ICD-9-CM is the US clinical modification of ICD-9 (Johns 2011, 237).

129. **b** ICD-9-CM is maintained by four organizations known as the cooperating parties: NCHS, the American Hospital Association (AHA), the American Health Information Management Association (AHIMA), and the Centers for Medicare and Medicaid Services (CMS). Primarily, NCHS is responsible for updating the diagnosis classification (Volumes 1 and 2), and CMS is responsible for updating the procedure classification (Volume 3). AHIMA works to help provide training and certification, and the AHA maintains the central office on ICD-9-CM and publishes *Coding Clinic for ICD-9-CM,* which contains the official coding guidelines and official guidance on the usage of ICD-9-CM codes (Johns 2011, 239).

130. **d** The most specific codes in the ICD-9-CM system are found at the subclassification level. Five-digit code numbers represent this level (Johns 2011, 240).

131. **d** Begin with the main term Revision; pacemaker site; chest (Kuehn 2012, 20, 27).

132. **c** Categories are further divided into subcategories. At this level, four-digit code numbers are used and the four-digit codes are referred to as subcategory codes (Johns 2011, 240).

133. **b** Begin with the main term Biopsy, artery, temporal (Kuehn 2012, 20, 27).

134. **b** E codes or external cause of injury codes, provide a means to classify environmental events, circumstances, and conditions as the cause of injury, poisoning, and other adverse effect. These codes are used in addition to codes from the main chapters of ICD-9-CM. E codes begin with the alpha character *E* and are followed by numerical characters (Johns 2011, 242).

135. **c** A query may not be appropriate because the clinical information or clinical picture does not appear to support the documentation of a condition or procedure. In situations where the provider's documented diagnosis does not appear to be supported by clinical findings, a healthcare entitiy's policies can provide guidance on a process for addressing the issue without querying the attending physician (Schraffenberger and Kuehn 2011, 348).

136. **a** The purpose of CPT is to provide a system for standard terminology and coding to report medical procedures and services provided by physicians and other clinical professionals. CPT is one of the most widely used systems for reporting medical services to health insurance carriers (Johns 2011, 255–256).

137. **d** Gunshot wounds, physical abuse, and substance abuse are not hospital-acquired conditions and therefore are not listed under the Hospital-Acquired Conditions Provision List (Casto and Layman 2011, 283–284).

138. **b** The quality of the documentation entered in the health record by providers can have major impacts on the ability of coding staff to perform their clinical analyses and assign accurate codes. In this situation, the best solution would be to educate the entire medical staff on their roles in the clinical documentation improvement process. Explaining to them the documentation guidelines and what documentation is needed in the record to support the more accurate coding of diabetes and its manifestations will reduce the need for coders to continue to query for this clarification (Schraffenberger and Kuehn 2011, 285).

139. **b** Validity is the degree to which codes accurately reflect the patient's diagnoses and procedures (Johns 2011, 266).

140. c A comorbid condition is a condition that existed at admission and is thought to increase the patient stay at least one day for approximately 75% of the patients. Diabetes existed at the time of admission (Johns 2011, 322).

141. a Given the examples, the geometric means are lower than the arithmetic means (Johns 2011, 323).

142. c Geographic practice cost index (GPCI) is the number used to multiply each relative value unit (RVU) so that it better reflects a geographical area's relative costs. The practice expense GPCI is higher in Seattle at 1.098 (Johns 2011, 326–327).

143. b 1.22 is the lowest relative value unit (Johns 2011, 327).

144. d Principal diagnosis is defined as the condition which, after study, is determined to have occasioned the admission of the patient to the hospital for care (Johns 2011, 319).

145. b In 1983, CMS implemented a PPS for inpatient hospital care provided to Medicare beneficiaries. This PPS methodology is called Medicare severity diagnosis-related groups (MS-DRGs). The MS-DRG system was implemented as a way to control Medicare spending. It reimburses hospitals a predetermined amount for each Medicare inpatient stay. Payments are determined by the MS-DRG to which each case is assigned according to the patient's principal diagnosis (Johns 2011, 321).

146. a To determine the appropriate MS-DRG, a claim for a healthcare encounter is first classified into one of 25 major diagnostic categories, or MDCs. The principal diagnosis determines the MDC assignment (Johns 2011, 322).

147. c To determine the appropriate MS-DRG, a claim for a healthcare encounter is first classified into one of 25 major diagnostic categories, or MDCs (Johns 2011, 322).

148. d NCCI is a predefined set of edits created by Medicare to prevent improper payment when incorrect code combinations are reported. The NCCI contains two tables of edits. The Column One/Column Two Correct Coding Edits table and the Mutually Exclusive Edits table include code pairs that should not be reported together for a number of reasons explained in the Coding Policy Manual (Schraffenberger and Kuehn 2011, 465).

149. b Medicare inpatients are reimbursed through MS-DRGs calculated for each hospital encounter. These are assigned with the help of a grouper (Casto and Layman 2011, 128).

150. d The importance of correct documentation to validate coding and ultimately billing cannot be overstated. Documentation must support the coding and billing (Brodnik et al. 2012, 432).

151. a Unbundling refers to a billing practice in which providers use multiple procedures code for a group of procedures instead of the appropriate combination code which may inappropriately maximize reimbursement (Brodnik et al. 2012, 443).

152. b Each base MS-DRG can be subdivided in one of three possible alternatives: MS-DRGs with three subgroups Major Complication/Comorbidity (MCC, CC, and non-CC); referred to as "with MCC," "with CC," and "w/o CC/MCC" (Johns 2011, 322).

153. **a** Present on admission (POA) is defined as a condition present at the time the order for inpatient admission occurs—conditions that develop during an outpatient encounter, including the emergency department, observation or outpatient surgery, are considered as present on admission. A POA indicator is assigned to principal and secondary diagnoses and the external cause of injury codes (Johns 2011, 325).

154. **a** Inpatient hospitals were required to submit POA information on diagnoses for inpatient Medicare discharges on or after October 1, 2007 (Johns 2011, 325).

155. **c** A major portion of HIPAA focused on identifying medically unnecessary services, upcoding, unbundling, and billing for services not provided. Unbundling is the practice of using multiple codes that describe individual components of a procedure rather than an appropriate single code that describes all steps of the procedure performed. Unbundling is a component of the NCCI and is what the coder in the example was doing. The use of audits and/or other evaluation techniques to monitor compliance and assist in the reduction of identified problem areas and corporate compliance is necessary to become aware of coding issues and stop those (Johns 2011, 358–359).

156. **b** CMS implemented the National Correct Coding Initiative (NCCI) in 1996 to develop correct coding methodologies to improve the appropriate payment of Medicare Part B claims (Johns 2011, 347).

157. **b** The NCCI edits (which most providers have built into their claims software) explain what procedures and services cannot be billed together on the same day of service for a patient. The mutually exclusive edit applies to improbable or impossible combinations of codes (Johns 2011, 347).

158. **a** The NCCI edits (which most providers have built into their claims software) explain what procedures and services cannot be billed together on the same day of service for a patient. The mutually exclusive edit applies to improbable or impossible combinations of codes (Johns 2011, 347–348).

159. **b** Coders should be evaluated at least quarterly, with appropriate training needs identified, facilitated, and reassessed over time. Only through this continuous process of evaluation can data quality and integrity be accurately measured and ensured (Schraffenberger and Kuehn 2011, 270).

160. **c** Quality coding is an important component of coding compliance. Standards for coding accuracy should be as close to 100% as possible (Schraffenberger and Kuehn 2011, 405).

161. **a** 385 charts per week / 5 days / 27 standard charts per day = 2.85 (Schraffenberger and Kuehn 2011, 276–279).

162. **c** Haldol is a drug frequently administered for behavior or mental conditions (Schraffenberger 2012, Appendix D, 9).

163. **b** There is a 72-hour window for Medicare patients. Outpatient and inpatient visits within the 72-hour period need to be reviewed to ensure complete and accurate coding and MS-DRG assignment (Schraffenberger and Kuehn 2011, 395–399).

164. **d** The error rates are not comparable since there are no data about the number of records coded during the period by each coder (Schraffenberger and Kuehn 2011, 319–320).

165. **c** A bronchoscopy with brushings and washings is considered a diagnostic bronchoscopy and not a biopsy. Code 31623 specifies brushings, and 31622 is selected for washings (Kuehn 2012, 136–137).

166. **a** MS-DRG sets exist where the listings of diagnoses used to drive the grouping are the same, but the presence or absence of a complication or comorbidity (CC) diagnosis or major complication or comorbidity (MCC) diagnosis assigns the case to a higher or lower MS-DRG. MS-DRG sets may contain to MS-DRGs or three MS-DRGs. These MS-DRG relationships and sets pose a compliance concern because the medical record documentation used to support the coding of principal diagnosis, complications, and comorbidities may not always be clear or used appropriately by the coder (such as undercoding). Therefore, inaccurate coding can lead to incorrect MS-DRG assignment and thus inappropriate reimbursement and can affect a hospital's case mix (Casto and Layman 2011, 45).

167. **b** The Fiscal Year 2009 Hospital-Acquired Conditions Provision List includes catheter-associated urinary tract infections; pressure ulcers; serious preventable event—object left in surgery, air embolism, blood incompatibility, vascular catheter-associated infections; mediastinitis after CABG, falls and fractures, dislocations, intracranial injury, crushing injuries, and burns (Casto and Layman 2011, 283–284).

168. **c** Treatment and anatomic location are not factors in the sequencing of burn conditions. Code all burns with the highest degree of burn sequenced first (Schraffenberger 2012, 363).

169. **b** Unlike hypertension and heart disease, ICD-9-CM presumes a cause-and-effect relationship between hypertension and chronic kidney disease, whether or not the condition is designated that way (Schraffenberger 2012, 183).

170. **a** AIDS stands for acquired immunodeficiency syndrome, frequently called human immunodeficiency infection. When a patient is treated for a complication associated with HIV infection, the 042 code is assigned as the principal diagnosis, followed by the code for the complication. Patients who are admitted for an HIV-related illness should be assigned a minimum of two codes in the following order: 042 to identify the HIV disease and additional codes to identify other diagnoses (Schraffenberger 2012, 83–84).

171. **c** Coding productivity is measured by two indicators of a coder's skill are the types of errors he or she makes and the speed at which he or she can work (Schraffenberger and Kuehn 2011, 76).

172. **d** AHA is responsible for issuing official advice via an editorial advisory board on behalf of the Cooperating Parties. Responses to coding questions posed by practitioners are published quarterly in *Coding Clinic for ICD-9-CM*. AMA maintains the CPT nomenclature system and publishes *CPT Assistant,* a monthly publication that communicates CPT guidelines and changes and that addresses CPT coding questions (Schraffenberger and Kuehn 2011, 15).

173. **a** In the acute-care setting, two main types of Medicare grouping programs are used: MS-DRGs for inpatient cases and APCs for outpatient cases (Schraffenberger and Kuehn 2011, 10).

174. **c** Any new coder should have 100% of his or her coded records reviewed prior to releasing the claim for quality review (Schraffenberger and Kuehn 2011, 353).

175. **c** The design and implementation of a data quality improvement program begin with setting the following goals: To establish ongoing monitor for identifying problems or developing opportunities to improve the quality of coded data; proactively identify variations in coding practice among staff members; determine the cause and scope of identified problems; set priorities for resolving identified problems; implement mechanisms to address and resolve issues identified; ensure corrective action for problems; implement a program to achieve compliance and also meet the needs of the organization (Schraffenberger and Kuehn 2011, 308).

176. **d** When the claim is submitted the reviewer should compare all the diagnoses and procedures printed on the bill with the coded information in the health record system. This process will help identify whether the communication software between the health record system and the billing system is functioning correctly. The HIM department should share the results of this comparison with patient financial services and the information technology department (Schraffenberger and Kuehn 2011, 320).

177. **d** MCC stands for major complications and comorbidities (Schraffenberger and Kuehn 2011, 201).

178. **b** If the treatment is directed at the malignancy, designate the malignancy as the principal diagnosis. The only exception to this guideline is if a patient admission or encounter is for the purpose of radiotherapy, immunotherapy, or chemotherapy. When the purpose of the encounter or hospital admission is for radiotherapy, or for antineoplastic chemotherapy, use the V code as the principal diagnosis (Schraffenberger 2012, 97–98).

179. **d** It is not appropriate for the coder to assume that the removal was done by either snare or hot biopsy forceps. The ablation code is only assigned when a lesion is completely destroyed and no specimen is retrieved. The coding professional must query the physician to assign the appropriate code (Schraffenberger and Kuehn 2011, 507).

180. **c** The patient had a normal delivery, full-term, single, healthy live born infant with an episiotomy. No other procedures or manipulation needed to aide in delivery (Schraffenberger 2012, 272–273).

181. **a** To move to a mature value-based purchasing program, CMS desires to pay for value—that is, to promote efficiency in resource use while providing high-quality care. To achieve this goal, CMS as a first step, established the hospital-acquired conditions provision in the acute-care inpatient setting (Casto and Layman, 2011, 283).

182. **d** HCPCS Level II codes were developed by CMS for use in reporting medical services not covered in CPT. Level II codes are provided for injectable drugs, ambulance services, prosthetic devices, and selected providers services. Crutches are classified as durable medical equipment and would be coded with a HCPCS Level II code (Smith 2012, 5).

183. **b** E codes, or external cause of injury codes, provide a means to classify environmental events, circumstances, and conditions as the cause of injury, poisoning, and other adverse effect. These codes must be used in addition to codes from the main chapters of ICD-9-CM. E codes begin with the alpha character *E* and are followed by numerical characters (Johns 2011, 242).

184. **a** Cardiac pacemakers are devices that send a small current through a lead (wire) to stimulate the heartbeat. There are two components to a pacemaker: generator (battery) and, attached to the generator, one or two leads (Smith 2012, 102).

185. **a**   Per CPT Coding Guidelines, when a planned procedure is terminated prior to completed for cause, the intended procedure is coded with a modifier. Because general anesthesia was used, modifier –74 is appropriate in this case (Schraffenberger and Kuehn, 2011, 53).

186. **c**   A healthcare entity's query policy should address the question of who to query. The query is directed to the provider who originated the progress note or other report in question. This could include the attending physician, consulting physician, or the surgeon. In most cases, a query for abnormal test results would be directed to the attending physician (Schraffenberger and Kuehn 2011, 44).

187. **d**   Queries are not necessary for every discrepancy or unaddressed issue in physician documentation. Healthcare entities should develop policies and procedures that clarify which clinical conditions and documentation situations warrant a request for physician clarification. Insignificant or irrelevant findings may not warrant a query regarding the assignment of an additional diagnosis code, for example. Entities must balance the value of collecting marginal data against the administrative burden of obtaining the additional documentation (Schraffenberger and Kuehn 2011, 44).

188. **d**   In fiscal year 2008 (October 1, 2007, through September 30, 2008), CMS developed the MS-DRG system to add a severity-adjustment component (Casto and Layman 2011, 121–122).

189. **b**   The outpatient code editor (OCE) operates in the systems of Medicare administrative contractors (MACs). The OCE provides a series of flags that can affect APC payments because it identifies coding errors in claims (Schraffenberger and Kuehn 2011, 209).

190. **c**   The National Correct Coding Initiative (NCCI or CCI) edits also apply to the APC system. The main purpose of CCI edits is to prohibit unbundling of procedures. CCI edits are updated quarterly (Schraffenberger and Kuehn 2011, 209).

191. **c**   Continuing education can be accomplished without sending staff to costly external seminars or workshops. The coding manager should consider the following few suggestions for internal continuing education (this is not a complete list): ask physicians from the medical staff to present short clinical topics pertinent to the patient population in a particular setting, have coders research pertinent clinical topics and make a presentation to their colleagues, and use resources available to you as a member of AHIMA. AHIMA provides a wealth of free resources in addition to low-cost alternatives, such as audio seminars, online courses, and the *CodeWrite* newsletter, that can be used to develop in-house coding training (Schraffenberger and Kuehn 2011, 58-59).

192. **b**   It is recommended that the healthcare entity's policy address the query format. A query generally includes the following information: patient name, admission date and/or date of service, health record number, account number, date query initiated, name and contact information of the individual initiating the query, and statement of the issue in the form of a question along with clinical indicators specified from the chart (e.g., history and physical states urosepsis, lab reports WBC of 14,400, emergency department report fever of 102°F) (Schraffenberger and Kuehn 2011, 45–46).

193. **b**   The record-over-record method of calculating errors considers each health record coded incorrectly as one error. The advantages of this method are that it allows for benchmarking with other hospitals that frequently use it, permits reviewers to track errors by case type, enables reviewers to relate productivity with quality errors on a case-by-case basis, and is much quicker to calculate. The disadvantages to this method are that it lacks specificity because it does not identify the coder's ability to assign codes that must be reported, and it does not identify the number of secondary diagnoses or procedures missed by the coder (Schraffenberger and Kuehn 2011, 319–320).

194. **c**   Often the consultant's report will identify specific issues or causes of coding variances that require further action. These items may include issuing queries to certain physicians to obtain additional information to modify the original coding, resubmitting claims to payers because the coding has been modified, discussing documentation deficiencies with one or more clinicians, addressing legibility issues with one or more physicians, and providing focused education to one or more coders. Another common error found includes duplicate codes (one from the coder assignment, also known as soft coding, and one from the CDM, also known as hard coding) This occurrence could cause duplicate payments by a payer and expose the organization to false billing allegations (Schraffenberger and Kuehn 2011, 324, 327).

195. **d**   Medical visits present several interesting aspects of the APC. For the most part, APCs follow the CPT coding rules as set forth by the AMA. However, for medical visits, hospitals have been able to develop their own criteria for assigning E/M codes that determine the level of the visit. In addition, hospitals do not follow the same guidelines as physicians (Schraffenberger and Kuehn 2011, 206).

196. **a**   The three components that make up the total RVU for a given procedure are physician work, practice expense, and malpractice expense (Schraffenberger and Kuehn 2011, 210).

197. **b**   The ICD-9-CM classification system often provides clues in the Alphabetic Index concerning the nature of a neoplasm. Adenocarcinoma is a known malignant neoplasm (Schraffenberger and Kuehn 2011, 443).

Domain III

198. **a**   The Outcomes and Assessment Information Set (OASIS-C) is a standardized data set designed to gather data about outcomes for Medicare beneficiaries who are receiving services from a home health agency (Johns 2011, 209).

199. **c**   A policy is a statement that describes general guidelines that direct behavior or direct and constrain decision making in the organization (Johns 2011, 460).

200. **b**   Fraudulent billing practices represent a major compliance risk for healthcare organizations. There are three of risk areas that are vitally important to the accuracy of the claims submission process: coding and billing, documentation, and medical necessity for tests and procedures. Areas within these three areas that are high risk billing practices include: billing for noncovered services, altered claim forms, duplicate billing, misrepresentation of facts on a claim form, failing to return overpayments, unbundling, billing for medically unnecessary services, overcoding and upcoding, billing for items or services not rendered, and false cost reports (Brodnik et al. 2012, 443–444).

1st : 51 / 80 = 64%

201. **a** The National Health Care Anti-Fraud Association defines healthcare fraud as an intentional deception or misrepresentation that the individual or entity makes knowing that the misrepresentation could result in some unauthorized benefit to the individual, or the entity or some other party. Healthcare abuse related to provider, supplier, and practitioner that are inconsistent with accepted sound fiscal, business, or medical practices with directly or indirectly result in: unnecessary costs to the program, false representation of a fact, damage to another party that reasonably relied on misrepresentation, failure to disclose a material fact, etc. (Brodnik et al. 2012, 430–431).

202. **b** The US Federal Sentencing Guidelines outline seven steps as the hallmark of an effective program to prevent and detect violations of law. These seven steps have become the blueprint for an effective compliance program for healthcare organizations (Brodnik et al. 2012, 450–451).

203. **a** There are a number of legal issues facing the EHR. State laws vary as to what is and is not acceptable in a court of law regarding EHRs. Healthcare providers frequently receive subpoenas requesting the production of the medical record. The subpoena may require the production of audit trails (Sayles and Trawick 2010, 264).

204. **a** Accreditation is the act of granting approval to a healthcare organization. The approval is base on whether the organization has met a set of voluntary standards that were developed by the accreditation agency. Voluntary reviews are conducted at the request of the healthcare facility seeking accreditation or certification. The Joint Commission is an example of an accreditation agency (Shaw and Elliott 2012, 330).

205. **b** The OIG has outlined seven elements as the minimum necessary for a comprehensive compliance program. One of the seven elements is the maintenance of a process, such as a hotline, to receive complaints and the adoption of procedures to protect the anonymity of complainants and to protect whistleblowers from retaliation (Johns 2011, 359).

206. **d** In conjunction with the corporate compliance officer, the health information manager should provide education and training related to the importance of complete and accurate coding, documentation and billing on an annual basis. Technical education for all coders should be provided. Documentation education is also part of compliance education. A focused effort should be made to provide documentation education to the medical staff (Schraffenberger and Kuehn 2011, 386–387).

207. **a** Within the federal government, the organization most involved in health services research is the Agency for Healthcare Research and Quality (AHRQ). AHRQ looks at issues related to the efficiency and effectiveness of the healthcare delivery system, disease protocols, and guidelines for improved disease outcomes (Johns 2011, 504).

208. **d** From February 1998 until the present, the OIG continues to issue compliance program guidance for various types of healthcare organizations. The OIG website (www.oig.hhs.gov) posts the documents that most healthcare organizations need to develop fraud and abuse compliance plans (Johns 2011, 359).

209. **a** Data security includes insuring that workstations are protected from unauthorized access. If a workstation is inactive for a period of time specified by the organization, it should log itself off automatically. The automatic log off helps prevent unauthorized users from accessing ePHI when an authorized user walks away from the computer without logging out of the system (Sayles and Trawick 2010, 316).

210. **c**   Retrospective utilization review is conducted after the patient has been discharged. Retrospective review examines the medical necessity of the services provided to the patient while in the hospital (Johns 2011, 651).

211. **b**   An EHR system can afford better security for PHI because authentication systems, access controls, audit logs, and other measures exist where they do not in a paper environment (Johns 2011, 184).

212. **a**   If physicians were to dictate information on patients they are treating in the facility, the disclosure of protected health information to the transcriptionists would be considered healthcare operations, and therefore, permitted under the HIPAA Privacy Rule. If physicians are dictating information on their private patients, however, it would be necessary for physicians to obtain a business associate agreement with the facility. It is permitted by the Privacy Rule for one covered entity to be a business associate of another covered entity (Thomason and Dennis 2008, 5).

213. **d**   The Joint Commission requires healthcare organizations to conduct in-depth investigations of occurrences that resulted—or could have resulted—in life-threatening injuries to patients, medical staff, visitors, and employees. The Joint Commission uses the *term sentinel* event for such occurrences (Johns 2011, 657–658).

214. **d**   Middle management is concerned primarily with facilitating the work performed by supervisory- and staff-level personnel as well as by executive leaders. The responsibilities of middle management include: developing, implementing, and revising the organization's policies and procedures under the direction of executive managers; executing the organizational plans developed at the board and executive levels; providing the operational information that executives need to develop meaningful plans for the organization's future (Johns 2011, 1024).

215. **a**   Staffing tools may be used to plan and manage staff resources. Staffing tools include: position descriptions outline the work and qualifications required by the job; performance standards establish expectations for how well the job will be done and how much work will be accomplished, written policies and procedures (discussed earlier) explaining staffing requirements and scheduling assist the supervisor in being fair and objective and help the staff understand the rules (Johns 2011, 1060).

216. **d**   The Joint Commission has been the most visible organization responsible for accrediting healthcare organizations since the mid-1950s. The primary focus of the Joint Commission at this time is to determine whether organizations seeking accreditation are continually monitoring the quality of the care they provide. The Joint Commission requires that this continual improvement process be in place throughout the entire organization, from the governing body down, as well as across all department lines (Shaw and Elliott 2012, 331).

217. **c**   A policy is a clearly stated and comprehensive statement that establishes the parameters for decision making and action. Policies are developed at both the institutional and departmental levels. In both cases, policies should be consistent within the organization. They must be developed in accordance with applicable laws and reflect actual practice (Johns 2011, 1031).

218. **c**   The Deficit Reduction Act of 2005 (DRA) was enacted in 2006. The DRA is particularly significant from a compliance perspective because it has transformed the nature of compliance programs from voluntary to mandatory (Brodnik et al. 2012, 439).

219. **b** Utilization review (UR) is the process of determining whether the medical care provided to a specific patient is necessary. Preestablished objective screening criteria are used as the basis of UR, which is performed according to time frames specified in the organizations UM plan (Johns 2011, 649–650).

220. **d** Types of utilization review include: preadmission review, continued-stay review and discharge review. Peer review is not a type of utilization review (Johns 2011, 650–651).

221. **c** Case management, discharge planning, and utilization review are all basic functions of the utilization review process; however, claims management is the process of managing the legal and administrative aspects of the healthcare organization's response to injury claims (Johns 2011, 649).

222. **d** To determine Joint Commission compliance, the rate of records completed within 30 days (or days specified in medical staff bylaws) must be computed. Average days are not the same as the rate of records delinquent (Joint Commission 2009).

223. **d** Since its beginning in 1952, TJC has continually evolved to meet the changing needs of healthcare organizations. Today, the Joint Commission is the largest healthcare standards-setting body in the world. It conducts accreditation surveys in more than 17,000 healthcare organizations and programs in the US (Johns 2011, 644).

224. **c** In this situation, the smaller hospital should obtain a business associate agreement with the facility providing the information services (Thomason and Dennis 2008, 2).

225. **b** To receive Medicare and Medicaid reimbursement, providers must prove that they follow the rules and regulations for participating in the Medicare program. Called the Medicare Conditions of Participation, these rules are set forth by CMS. Facilities that must meet the standards in the Conditions of Participation include hospitals, home health agencies, ambulatory surgical centers, and hospices (Johns 2011, 721–722).

226. **a** Auditing information system activity is an important part of a data security program. Auditing provides a means of identifying potential access and other abuses. Auditing of an information system is performed by examining and evaluating audit trails. An audit trail is a record of system and application activity by users. It can track when an employee has accessed the system and how long the employee has been logged into a system (Johns 2011, 926).

227. **a** Beginning with its acute hospital standards in 2004, the Joint Commission initiated a new process that moved from survey monitors every three years to a philosophy of continuous improvement and continuous standard compliance. Standards were streamlined and survey paperwork reduced, facility monitoring of sentinel (unexpected) events was encouraged, and following the hospital experience of selected patients (tracer methodology) during its surveys was instituted. Each accreditation standard was accompanied by a rationale and steps to meet the standard, called elements of performance (Johns 2011, 110).

228. **d** The Healthcare Quality Improvement Act established the National Practitioner Data Bank (NPDB). The purpose of the NPDB is to provide a clearinghouse for information about medical practitioners who have a history of malpractice suits and other quality problems. Hospitals are required to consult the NPDB before granting medical staff privileges to healthcare practitioners (Johns 2011, 691).

229. **b** The medical staff operates according to a predetermined set of policies called the medical staff bylaws. The bylaws spell out the specific qualifications that physicians must demonstrate before they can practice medicine in the hospital. They are considered legally binding. Any changes to the bylaws must be approved by a vote of the medical staff and the hospital's governing body (Johns 2011, 711).

230. **b** The leader of the administrative staff is the CEO or chief administrator. The CEO is responsible for implementing the policies and strategic direction set by the hospital's board of directors. He or she also is responsible for building an effective executive management team and coordinating the hospital's services (Johns 2011, 711).

231. **d** Today, medical school graduates must pass a test before they can obtain a license to practice medicine. The licensure tests are administered by state medical boards. Many states now use a standardized licensure test developed in 1968 by the Federation of State Medical Boards of the United States. However, passing scores for the test vary by state. Most physicians also complete several years of residency training in addition to medical school (Johns 2011, 676).

232. **b** Section 164.524 of the Privacy Rule states that an individual has a right of access to inspect and obtain a copy of his or her own PHI that is contained in a designated record set, such as a health record. The individual's right extends for as long as the PHI is maintained. However, there are exceptions to what PHI may be accessed. For example, psychotherapy notes; information compiled in reasonable anticipation of a civil, criminal, or administrative action or proceeding; or PHI subject to the Clinical Laboratory Improvements Act (CLIA) are all exceptions (Johns 2011, 826–827).

233. **c** The HIPAA Privacy Rule provides patients with significant rights that allow them to have some measure of control over their health information. As long as state laws or regulations or the physician does not state otherwise, competent adult patients have the right to access their health record (Brodnik et al. 2012, 241).

234. **b** HIPAA allows the covered entity to impose a reasonable cost-based fee when the individual requests a copy of PHI or agrees to accept summary or explanatory information. The fee may include the cost of: copying, including supplies and labor; postage, when the individual has requested that the copy or summary or explanation be mailed; preparing an explanation or summary, if agreed to by the individual. HIPAA does not permit "retrieval fees" to be charged to patients. However, they are permitted for nonpatient requests (Johns 2011, 831).

☆ 235. **d** One strategy included in a good security program is an employee security awareness program. Employees are often responsible for threats to data security. Consequently, employee awareness is a particularly important tool in reducing security breaches (Johns 2011, 992).

☆ 236. **a** Within the context of data security, protecting data *privacy* basically means defending of safeguarding access to information. Only those individuals who need to know information should be authorized to access it (Johns 2011, 984).

237. **b** Data security can be defined as the protection measures and tools for safeguarding information and information systems (Johns 2011, 982–983).

238. **c** The HIPAA Privacy Rule intent is to allow an individual to obtain copies of records for a fee that is reasonable enough that an individual could pay for it. The Privacy Rule requires that the copy fee for the individual be reasonable and cost based. It can only include the costs of labor for copying, and postage, when mailed. The commentary to the Privacy Rule expands upon this standard. If paper copies are made, the fee can include the cost of the paper. If electronic copies are made, the fee can include copies of the media used (Thomason and Dennis 2008, 82).

239. **a** Risk management begins by conducting a risk analysis. Identifying security threats or risks, determining how likely it is that any given threat may occur, and estimating the impact of an untoward event are all parts of a risk assessment (Johns 2011, 989).

240. **a** HIPAA requires that organizations establish a written contingency plan to be developed and tested. This is to ensure that procedures are in place to handle an emergency response in the event of an untoward event (Johns 2011, 1002–1003).

241. **D** HIPAA requires covered entities to maintain their security measures. The administrative provisions detail how the security program should be managed from the organization's perspective. Policies and procedures should be written and formalized in a policy manual. The organization should issue a statement of its philosophy on data security. Further, it should make a chart outlining data security authority and responsibilities throughout the organization (Johns 2011, 1001–1002).

242. **c** Employees are the biggest threat to the security of healthcare data. Whether it is disgruntled employees destroying computer hardware, snooping employees accessing information without authorization to do so, or employees accessing information for fraudulent purposes, employees are a real threat to data security (Johns 2011, 987).

243. **b** All data security policies and procedures should be reviewed and evaluated at least every year to make sure they are up-to-date and still relevant to the organization (Johns 2011, 995).

244. **c** Good forms design is needed within an EHR to create ease of use. The use of a selection box allows the user to select a value from a predefined list. Check boxes are used for multiple selections and radio buttons are used for single selections (Johns 2011, 440).

245. **d** Every healthcare organization should have a forms or design (for EHR systems) committee. The medical records committee also may function in this capacity. This committee should provide oversight for the development, review, and control of all enterprise-wide information capture tools, including paper forms and design of computer screens (Johns 2011, 415–416).

246. **d** Utilization review is the process of determining whether the medical care provided to a specific patient is necessary according to preestablished objective screening criteria (Johns 2011, 1179).

247. **c** Physical access controls are safeguards that protect physical equipment, media, or facilities. For example, doors leading to the areas that house mainframes and other principal computing equipment should have locks on them. In addition, locks should be installed on personal computers and terminals to help guard against theft. Other physical controls might include positioning computer terminal screens so that confidential data are not exposed to public view (Johns 2011, 992).

248. **a** Paper ranging from 20 to 24 lb. is recommended for use in copiers, scanners, and fax machines. In an EDMS, paper forms are added to the electronic medical record via a scanner so the weight of the paper is important (Johns 2011, 415).

249. **c** Determination if a breach has occurred should be completed before action is taken. The audit trail is a software program that tracks every single access to data in the computer system. It logs the name of the individual who accessed the data, the date and time, and the action taken (for example, modifying, reading, or deleting data). Depending on the organization's policy, audit trails are reviewed periodically or on predetermined schedules. Audit trails document when data have been accessed and by whom. Review of audit trails can help detect whether a breach of security has occurred (Johns 2011, 993).

250. **c** Coding policies should include the following components: AHIMA Code of Ethics, AHIMA Standards of Ethical Coding, Official Coding Guidelines, applicable federal and state regulations, internal documentation policies requiring the presence of physician documentation to support all coded diagnosis and procedure code assignments (Schraffenberger and Kuehn 2011, 384).

251. **b** Title II of HIPAA mandated the establishment of fraud and abuse control programs to battle healthcare fraud and abuse. Monies were appropriated to fund those programs, and agencies were identified to participate in the government's efforts. Additionally, the Medicare Integrity Program was established. This program was charged with the following responsibilities: review of provider activities for potential fraudulent activity, audit of cost reports, payment determinations, education of providers and beneficiaries on healthcare fraud and abuse issues (Schraffenberger and Kuehn 2011, 372).

252. **a** Access to ePHI can be controlled through the use of the following: user-based access, role-based access, and context-based access. Role-based access control decisions are based on the roles individual users have as part of an organization. Each user is given various privileges to perform their role or function (Brodnik et al. 2012, 304).

253. **a** Review of records by the patient is permitted after the authorization for use and disclosure is verified. Usually hospital personnel should be present during on-site reviews to assist the requester with the paper record or working with the EHR if necessary. Assistance would not be needed if the people requesting on-site review work for the facility (Brodnik et. al. 2012, 358–359).

254. **c** The HIPAA Privacy Rule provides patients with significant rights that allow them to have some measure of control over their health information. As long as state laws or regulations or the physician does not state otherwise, competent adult patients have the right to access their health record (Brodnik et al. 2012, 240).

255. **c** Because HIPAA defers to state laws on the issue of minors, applicable state laws should be consulted regarding appropriate authorization. In general, the age of maturity is 18 years or older. This is the legal recognition that an individual is considered responsible for, and has control over, his or her actions (Brodnik et al. 2012, 154).

256. **b** Fraudulent billing practices represent a major compliance risk for healthcare organizations. There are three of risk areas that are vitally important to the accuracy of the claims submission process: coding and billing, documentation, and medical necessity for tests and procedures. Areas within these three areas that are high-risk billing practices include billing for non-covered services, altered claim forms, duplicate billing, misrepresentation of facts on a claim form, failing to return overpayments, unbundling, billing for medically unnecessary services, overcoding and upcoding (thus ignoring official coding guidelines), billing for items or services not rendered, and false cost reports (Brodnik et al. 2012, 441–445).

257. **a**   Called the Medicare Conditions of Participation, these rules are set forth by CMS. Facilities that must meet the standards in the Conditions of Participation include hospitals, home health agencies, ambulatory surgical centers, and hospices (Johns 2011, 722).

258. **a**   The nationwide expansion of RAC was to be fully implemented and operational by January 2010 (Schraffenberger and Kuehn 2011, 376).

259. **c**   Single sign-on enables sign-on to multiple related, but independent, software systems. With this property a user logs in once and gains access to all systems without being prompted to log in again at each of them. Single sign-off is the reverse property whereby a single action of signing out terminates access to multiple software systems (Johns 2011, 921).

260. **c**   Physical access controls are safeguards that protect physical equipment, media, or facilities. For example, doors leading to the areas that house mainframes and other principal computing equipment should have locks on them. In addition, locks should be installed on personal computers and terminals to help guard against theft. Other physical controls might include positioning computer terminal screens so that confidential data are not exposed to public view (Johns 2011, 992).

261. **b**   The term *access control* means being able to identify which employees should have access to what data. The general practice is that employees should have access only to data they need to do their jobs. For example, an admitting clerk and a healthcare provider would not have access to the same kinds of data (Johns 2011, 992).

262. **b**   The audit trail is a software program that tracks every single access to data in the computer system. It logs the name of the individual who accessed the data, the date and time, and the action taken (for example, modifying, reading, or deleting data). Depending on the organization's policy, audit trails are reviewed periodically or on predetermined schedules. Audit trails document when data have been accessed and by whom. Review of audit trails can help detect whether a breach of security has occurred (Johns 2011, 993).

263. **c**   The three steps in medical necessity and utilization review are: clinical review, peer review, and appeals consideration (Casto and Layman 2011, 99).

264. **a**   Managers must stay up-to-date on compliance issues that are published and discussed in various government and other third-party payer documents. The OIG workplan should be reviewed each year. This document provides insight into the directions the OIG is taking, as well as highlights hot areas of compliance (Casto Layman 2011, 43).

265. **d**   In Medicare the most common forms of fraud and abuse include billing for services not furnished; misrepresenting the diagnosis to justify payment; soliciting, offering, or receiving a kickback, unbundling, falsifying certificates of medical necessity, and billing for a service not furnished as billed, known as upcoding (Casto and Layman 2011, 35).

266. **b**   Managed care systems control costs primarily by presetting payment amounts and restricting patient access to healthcare services through precertification and utilization review processes (Johns 2011, 718).

267. **d** The policies and procedures section of a Coding Compliance Plan should include physician query process, coding diagnosis not supported by medical documentation, upcoding, correct use of encoder software, unbundling, coding medical records without complete documentation, assignment of discharge destination codes, and complete process for using scrubber software. Utilization review would not be part of the policies and procedures section of a Coding Compliance Plan (Casto and Layman 2011, 42).

268. **c** Evidence-based clinical practice guidelines are the foundation of members' care for specific clinical conditions. Evidence-based clinical practice guidelines are explicit statements that guide clinical decision making (Casto and Layman 2011, 98).

269. **a** The gatekeeper role of the primary care provider is cost control. Gatekeepers determine the appropriateness of the healthcare service, the level of healthcare personnel, and the setting in the continuum of care (Casto and Layman 2011, 100).

270. **c** A common theme runs through safe harbors and that is the intent to protect certain arrangements in which commercially reasonable items or services are exchanged for fair market value compensation. Safe harbors are an exception to the Federal Anti-Kickback Statute. Congress authorized HHS to establish additional safe harbors by regulation. These safe harbors are activities that are not subject to prosecution and protect the organization from civil or criminal penalties (Brodnik et al. 2012, 436–437).

271. **b** The emergency operations plan is practiced twice a year in response either to an actual disaster or to a planned drill. Exercises should stress the limits of the organization's emergency management system to assess preparedness capabilities and performance when systems are stressed (Shaw and Elliott 2012, 262).

272. **a** The Commission on Accreditation of Rehabilitation Facilities (CARF) is a private, not-for-profit organization committed to developing and maintaining practical, customer-focused standards to help organizations measure and improve the quality, value, and outcomes of behavioral health and medical rehabilitation programs. CARF accreditation is based on an organization's commitment to continually enhance the quality of its services and programs and to focus on customer satisfaction (Shaw and Elliott 2012, 332).

273. **a** Hospitals accredited through the Joint Commission or other accrediting body may participate in the Medicare program because the accrediting agency has been granted deemed status by the Medicare program. Deemed status means accrediting bodies such as the Joint Commission can survey facilities for compliance with the Medicare Conditions of Participation for Hospitals instead of the government (Odom-Wesley et al. 2009, 291).

274. **c** The Joint Commission uses tracer methodology for on-site surveys. The tracer methodology incorporates the use of the priority focus process (PFP) review, follows the experience of care through the organization's entire healthcare process and allows the surveyor to identify performance issues (Odom-Wesley et al. 2009, 305–306).

275. **d** Services that are cosmetic, elective, and investigational are much less likely to be considered medically necessary. Standard of care for health condition would be much more likely to be considered medically necessary (Casto and Layman 2011, 99–100).

276. **c** Goals of case management include continuity of care, cost-effectiveness, quality, and appropriate utilization (Casto and Layman 2011, 101).

277. **b** An Advance Beneficiary Notice (ABN) should be provided to a patient when a service is not considered medically necessary indicating that Medicare might not pay and that the patient may be responsible for the entire charge (Schraffenberger and Kuehn 2011, 396).

DOMAIN IV
46/64 = 72%

278. **a** The health record number is important because it uniquely identifies not only the patient, but also the patient's record. Patient care documentation generated as part of the patient's episode of care is identified and physically filed or linked in an electronic system. Social security numbers (SSNs) have been proposed for use as a unique patient identification number; however, the Social Security Administration is adamant in its opposition to using the SSN for purposes other than those identified by law. The American Health Information Management Association (AHIMA) is in agreement on this issue due to privacy, confidentiality, and security issues related to the use of the SSN (Johns 2011, 387).

279. **d** Unified messaging is the ability for an individual to receive and/or retrieve various forms of messaging at a single access point, including voice, e-mail, fax, and video mail (Johns 2011, 1177).

280. **d** The chief information officer (CIO) is a senior-level executive. He or she is responsible for leading the strategic IS planning process, for assisting the leadership team to use IS in support of strategic planning and management, and for overseeing the organization's IRM functions. These functions are performed by the IS department as well as by the telecommunications, management engineering, and HIM departments. The CIO typically reports directly to the organization's chief executive officer (CEO) (Johns 2011, 963).

281. **c** As the electronic system develops, different versions of documents may exist and these also must be monitored and logged for both legal and practice purposes. Additionally, the AHIMA e-HIM Task Force (AHIMA 2004) describes in detail changes in health information processes and procedures that are required as a record transitions from paper to hybrid to fully electronic formats (Johns 2011, 123).

282. **d** Data must be available continuously. When paper as a backup no longer exists in a paperless EHR environment, users must be assured that the computer system is available to them at all times. To achieve such availability, an EHR should have server redundancy accomplished through mirrored processing. This means that as data are entered and processed by one server, they are entered and processed simultaneously by a second server. Should the primary server crash, the system should be designed to "fail over" to the second server and can continue processing as if, at least from the user's point of view, nothing had happened (Johns 2011, 169).

283. **c** In an attempt to get as much medical record information online as possible, many hospitals turned to document imaging and COLD (computer output to laser disk) systems. Document imaging systems involve scanning documents created on paper and making their images available on a computer monitor. COLD systems capture print images of lab results and other documents that are in stand-alone electronic systems and make them available for viewing on a computer monitor. Because of the use of newer storage media, COLD systems are more commonly referred to as electronic (or enterprise) report management (ERM) systems (Johns 2011, 143).

284. **b** Today, EHR systems are generally based on the use of a clinical data repository (CDR), a special kind of database that manages data from different source systems in the hospital or other provider settings, including direct entry of discrete data by the clinician. CDRs can process discrete data from various ancillary systems, such as laboratory, pharmacy, and radiology systems. They also can store and make accessible paper document images and clinical images such as those from PACS (Johns 2011, 144).

285. **b** The vocabulary used in an EHR system should, at a minimum, be a controlled vocabulary. A controlled vocabulary means that a specific set of terms in the EHR's data dictionary may be used and that a central authority approves any additions or changes. A controlled vocabulary is essential to ensure common meaning for all users (Johns 2011, 162).

286. **d** Many hospitals begin their EHR implementation with point of care (POC) charting systems. These systems provide context-sensitive templates. Templates ensure that the appropriate data are collected and guide users in adhering to professional practice standards. These might include nursing admission assessments, nursing progress notes, vital signs charting, intake/output records, and the like (Johns 2011, 145).

287. **c** Document imaging systems have become more sophisticated and today are called electronic document management systems (EDMSs). They can manage many types of digital documents, including e-mails and electronic faxes. When EDMSs are well indexed, certain content within the documents can be uniquely retrieved (Johns 2011, 143–144).

288. **c** Computerized provider order entry (CPOE) is an application that uses standard order sets and other CDS that supports physician order entry into the computer. As the orders are entered, physicians get immediate feedback from CDS systems as to whether there are drug contraindications, what the appropriate protocol is for diagnostic studies, when to provide preventative care services or screenings, and so on. Once the physician signs off on the orders they are automatically routed to their respective destinations (for example, lab orders to the laboratory information system, drug orders to the pharmacy information system, diet orders to food and nutrition services information system) (Johns 2011, 146).

289. **d** The unique identifier in the patient table is the patient number. It is unique to each patient. Patient last name, first name, and date of birth can be shared with other patients, but the identifier will not (Johns 2011, 903–904)

290. **b** Due diligence involves thoroughly reviewing the vendors' proposals, conducting product demonstrations, visiting sites where the product is already installed, calling references, and investigating the vendors' business practices. The organization must be assured that not only will the EHR function as expected, but that the vendor will do a good job implementing it, provide appropriate support when there are problems, keep it current, and remain in business (Johns 2011, 172, 177).

291. **c** The paper-based record assembly process described earlier is replaced by record preparation and document scanning in the hybrid and EHR environment. Records are prepared for scanning by repairing torn forms, removing staples, and adding header forms to the front of the records. Additionally, checks are made to ensure that all pages are identified accurately as part of the individual patient's record (Johns 2011, 422).

292. **a** An implementation plan is a much more detailed plan that identifies what often is hundreds, if not thousands, of steps to implement each application. The vendor usually supplies a generic plan for how it likes to implement the EHR. It is important to adjust the vendor's plan outlining implementation details with the organization's plan, which will include some of the same and additional tasks (Johns 2011, 178).

293. **a** Computerized provider order entry (CPOE) is an application that uses standard order sets and other CDS that supports physician order entry into the computer. As the orders are entered, physicians get immediate feedback from CDS systems as to whether there are drug contraindications, what the appropriate protocol is for diagnostic studies, when to provide preventative care services or screenings, and so on. Once the physician signs off on the orders, they are automatically routed to their respective destinations (Johns 2011, 146–147).

294. **d** There are important applications that support EHR functionality. Many hospitals begin their EHR implementation with POC charting systems. These systems provide context-sensitive templates. Templates ensure that the appropriate data are collected and guide users in adhering to professional practice standards. These might include nursing admission assessments, nursing progress notes, vital signs charting, intake/output records, and the like (Johns 2011, 145).

295. **c** Relations are established in a relational database by the primary key of one table becoming a foreign key in another table. In this case, patient # is the primary key in the patient table and used as the foreign key in the visit table (Johns 2011, 158–159, 903–904).

296. **b** It is critical to provide adequate training for the end-users of a new information system. For any new system to be successful, it must be accepted and used by the staff. When the staff is not thoroughly trained, the result may be low morale and dissatisfaction with the system (Johns 2011, 890–891).

297. **b** User-based access is a security mechanism used to grant users of a system access based on the identity of the user (Brodnik et al. 2012, 304).

298. **d** A portal is a special application to provide secure remote access to specific applications (Johns 2011, 137).

299. **a** Client/server (C/S) architecture uses a combination of computers to capture and process data. Server computers are powerful processors. They typically house all the application software and store all active data captured by all the clients throughout the network. They then "serve" multiple client computers, which have less powerful processors (and in some cases have minimal processing capability of their own, in which case they are called thin clients) (Johns 2011, 167).

300. **c** Interoperability refers to the use of standard protocols to enable two different computer systems to share data with each other (Johns 2011, 153).

301. **a** The long-term goal of the transaction standards is to allow providers and plans or payers to seamlessly transfer data back and forth with little intervention. To do this, HHS adopted the electronic transaction standards of ASC X12 Insurance Subcommittee (Accredited Standards Committee Health Care Task group (X12N). The standards adopted for EDI are called ANSI ASC X12N (Johns 2011, 219).

302. **a** Health records are used for a number of purposes related to patient care. The primary purposes of the health record are associated directly with the provision of patient care services (Johns 2011, 34).

303. **d** To take advantage of CDS much of the information in the EHR must be captured in discrete data format (also referred to as structured data) from ancillary systems or from data entered by the clinician and/or patient using templates and other data entry aids. Discrete data consists of data elements that are raw facts or figures that can be processed by the computer (Johns 2011, 139).

304. **c** In general, an HIE organization requires some specific form of governance, policies and procedures for exchanging health information, security utilities, identity matching algorithm, and record locator service (RLS). Because the US does not have a national patient identifier, an identity matching algorithm process must be used by HIE organizations to identify any patient for whom data are to be exchanged. This algorithm uses sophisticated probability equations to identify patients (Johns 2011, 151).

305. **a** Today, EHR systems are generally based on the use of a clinical data repository (CDR), a special kind of database that manages data from different source systems in the hospital or other provider settings, including direct entry of discrete data by the clinician. CDRs can process discrete data from various ancillary systems, such as laboratory, pharmacy, and radiology systems. They also can store and make accessible paper document images and clinical images such as those from PACS (Johns 2011, 144).

306. **d** Computerized provider order entry (CPOE) is an application that uses standard order sets and other CDS that supports physician order entry into the computer. As the orders are entered, physicians get immediate feedback from CDS systems as to whether there are drug contraindications, what the appropriate protocol is for diagnostic studies, when to provide preventative care services or screenings, and so on. Once the physician signs off on the orders they are automatically routed to their respective destinations (Johns 2011, 146).

307. **a** Workflow support also has been added to EDMSs. This means that the EDMS facilitates various functions that must be performed, often simultaneously or in a specific sequence (Johns 2011, 143, 164).

308. **c** A mainframe is a computer architecture built with a single central processing unit to which dumb terminals and/or personal computers are connected. Mainframes were the only computers available until the late 1960s. They can perform millions of instructions per second, are designed to connect input/output devices over long distances and can handle hundreds or thousands of users at the same time (Johns 2011, 894).

309. **b** When EDMSs are well indexed, certain content within the documents can be uniquely retrieved making EDMS a good transition for the healthcare organization on their way to a fully interactive EHR (Johns 2011, 143).

310. **c** Many organizations find that their HIS vendor does not provide the level of EHR sophistication they desire and are looking to interface their HIS applications with clinical applications from another vendor. Sometimes called dual core, in this vendor strategy one vendor primarily supplies the financial and administrative applications and another vendor primarily supplies the clinical applications (Johns 2011, 176).

311. **d** Essentially, a document imaging system scans and indexes an original source document to create a digital picture that can be retrieved via the computer. When scanned, the images are stored on electronic media, such as a magnetic or optical disk. Unlike microfilm rolls, the optical disk is a random-access device and retrieval of documents is much faster. Additionally, document images can be viewed by more than one person at one time and at different locations. One of the greatest benefits of document imaging is increased efficiency by eliminating the requirement to move and track paper documents through workflow. Document imaging also helps solve the problem of lost or misplaced paper or microfiche documents (Johns 2011, 401).

312. **d** A transaction-processing system (TPS) is an example of an operations support system. A TPS manages the different kinds of transactions that occur in a healthcare facility. Patient admissions, employee time cards, and supply purchases are examples of transactions that take place in a healthcare facility (Johns 2011, 878).

313. **d** Information systems must be created in a logical manner. The system development life cycle (SDLC) is the traditional way to plan and implement an IS in an organization. The major phases of the cycle are planning, analysis, design, implementation, and maintenance (Johns 2011, 882–883).

314. **c** To understand the nature of a computer network, it is important to first understand the nature of communications systems. A communications system is made up of four components: a transmitter, a receiver, the medium, and data (Johns 2011, 911).

315. **a** Interoperability allows information to be shared from one computer system with another. This sharing of information along with standardization is necessary for all of the systems to work together, thus providing us with a seamless integration of data (Johns 2011, 953).

316. **c** The request for proposal (RFP) is a written document that generally includes a detailed description of the requirements for the system and gives guidelines for vendors to follow in bidding for the contract (Johns 2011, 889).

317. **b** The *direct cutover approach,* the organization stops using the old system and starts the new one on a specified date. This approach is risky, but can work effectively when sufficient testing was done and adequate backup procedures are in place. In fact, it may make more sense to convert via the direct cutover method when the old system is quite different from the new one (Johns 2011, 891).

318. **d** Given the size and complexity of healthcare organizations and the number of emerging technologies, strategic information system planning is an essential first step in adopting new IS technology. Strategic information systems planning is the process of identifying and assigning priorities to the various upgrades and changes that might be made in an organization's information systems (Johns 2011, 883–884).

319. **b** The implementation phase is a complex undertaking and includes the development of the computer programs, testing of the system, and development of system documentation, user training, and system conversion. Typically, the organization designates an interdisciplinary implementation team led by a project manager to develop a plan for implementing the new system (Johns 2011, 888).

320. **d** The personal health record (PHR) is a relatively new concept that encourages patients to take an active role in their health information. AHIMA defines the PHR as an electronic, universally available, lifelong resource of health information needed by individuals to make health decisions. Patients are expected to own and manage the information in the PHR, which comes from both healthcare providers and the individual (Johns 2011, 155).

321. **d** The idea of allowing patient-generated data into the EHR is also emerging. Some organizations support a patient portal where the patients may log on to a website from home or a kiosk in a provider's waiting room to schedule appointments, pay bills, obtain patient educational material, sign informed consents, request release of information, enter health history data using a context-specific template, or even engage in an e-visit, which is now reimbursable by some insurance companies (Johns 2011, 155).

322. **c**   An alert notifies a physician of a potential contraindication. For example, the attending physician recommended that Mrs. Mason be admitted immediately. He also ordered a cardiac catheterization and several medications. The cardiac catheterization laboratory was notified of the admission, and the procedure was scheduled through the hospital's scheduling system. The pharmacy component of the hospital's IS alerted the physician to a possible drug interaction. In response to the pharmacy alert, the physician altered his medication order for Mrs. Mason (Johns 2011, 951).

323. **c**   An MIS is supported by TPS data to help middle managers make decisions about their departments' objectives. MISs are usually specialized, designed to support a particular area of the business. In an HIM MIS, for example, input data might include admission, discharge, and transfer data; and data on the number of dictated reports, coded records, filed records, and incomplete records. Examples of the outputs would include structured reports, production schedules, and productivity analysis so that the HIM Director can make management decisions (Johns 2011, 879–880).

324. **a**   The principal purpose of the data warehouse is to provide data for improved decision support. A data warehouse usually contains historical data that is derived from operation (transaction) systems and is optimized for speed of retrieval of data, thus enhancing decision making (Johns 2011, 158, 909).

325. **c**   An expert system (ES) is a knowledge system built from a set of rules applied to specific problems. It can take the place of a human expert when it comes to problem solving. The system simulates the reasoning process of human experts in certain well-defined areas (Johns 2011, 881).

326. **b**   A relational database stores data in predefined tables that contain rows and columns similar to a spreadsheet. The kinds of data that can be stored in a relational database are currency, real numbers, integers, and strings (characters of data). This type of database is a popular model used in healthcare applications (Johns 2011, 902–903).

327. **d**   Primary keys ensure that each row in a table is unique. A primary key must not change in value. Typically, a primary key is a number that is a one-up counter or a randomly generated number in large databases (Johns 2011, 903).

328. **c**   The purpose of a database is to store and retrieve data. A popular common language called structured query language (SQL) is used to store and retrieve data in relational databases (Johns 2011, 902).

329. **a**   Data models provide a contextual framework and graphical representation that aid in the definition of data elements (Johns 2011, 904).

330. **d**   One common approach to staff training is a train-the-trainer program. In this approach, key people in the various functional areas are identified and trained first. They then train the other users in their area. This approach is effective because the trainers are still available to help the staff after the system has been installed and the vendor is no longer on-site to answer questions (Johns 2011, 891).

331. **a**   The purpose of a network is to allow users to share its resources easily and efficiently. For example, any network user can access the network printer, not just the user sitting behind the computer to which the printer is attached (Johns 2011, 911–912).

332. c   In an AHIMA Practice Brief, Walsh (2011) recommends a system that uses a two-factor authentication. He identifies three methods for authentication—any combination of two of these would constitute a two-factor system. The three methods are something you know such as a password or PIN; something you have, such as an ATM card, token, or swipe, smart card; and something you are, such as a biometric fingerprint, voice scan, iris, or retinal scan (Brodnik et al. 2012, 305).

333. c   Data must be available continuously. To achieve such availability, an EHR should have a server redundancy. This means that as data are entered and processed by one server, they are entered and processed simultaneously by a second server. Should the primary server crash, the system should be designed to "fail-over" to the second server and continue processing as if nothing had happened (Johns, 2011, 169).

334. a   Results retrieval technology maybe as basic as a look-up where a query is made to access certain data from a specific system. Navigational tools permit the user to select a specific data element, make a customized table, or graph results (Johns 2011, 164).

335. b   An important element in planning and implementation is addressing issues management. Issues will always arise. For example, hardware may not be delivered on time, a server may be delivered dead on arrival, and a system may be not be fixed correctly the first time. An issues log should be maintained to ensure that every issue is resolved (Johns 2011, 178).

336. a   An EHR includes a considerable amount of electronic information that is created as a byproduct of the software and is not a part of the user-entered information. Metadata includes data and file attributes, audit logs, software code, temporary information such as "sticky-notes" and alert pop-ups. Obviously these are not part of the paper medical record and so would not be part of what should be disclosed under routine subpoenas or court orders for EHRs (Johns 2011, 186).

337. c   Health Level Seven (HL7), founded in 1987, is a not-for-profit, ANSI-accredited standards developing organization that provides comprehensive standards for the exchange, integration, sharing, and retrieving of electronic health information that supports patient care..The HL7 standard allows exchange of data between common systems that make up the EHR such as radiology, laboratory, pharmacy, and other systems. HL7 is a family of standards that aid the exchange of data among hospital systems and, more recently, physician practices and other types of provider systems (Johns 2011, 916–917).

338. a   The data element PATIENT_LAST_NAME must be stored as character data because the data are character-based (Johns 2011, 906–907).

339. c   Thorough testing of new systems (hardware and/or software) before the actual conversion date is critical. Systems testers test the use cases developed in the design phase against the system's requirements. Testing should be conducted using actual patient data, not sample data the vendor has provided or the organization has created for training purposes. Correcting a problem in the test mode is often easier than correcting it after the system is fully operational (Johns 2011, 890).

340. d   A foreign key is a column of one table that corresponds to a primary key in another table. Together, they allow two tables to join together (Johns 2011, 903).

341. c   One security strategy is to implement application controls. These are controls contained in the application software or computer programs. One common application control is password management. It involves keeping a record of end users' identifications and passwords and then matching the passwords to each end user's privileges (Johns 2011, 992).

342. **c** In the HIPAA Security Rule, one of the technical safeguards standards is access control. This includes automatic log-off, which ensure electronic processes that terminate an electronic session after a predetermined time of inactivity (Brodnik et al. 2012, 307).

Domain V 343. **a** Digital scanners create images of handwritten and printed documents that are then store in health record databases as electronic files. The data can be interfaced in the current EHR with the document scanning system. Using scanned images solves many of the problems associated with traditional paper-based health records and hybrid records (Odom-Wesley et al. 2009, 227).

344. **b** Aspiration pneumonia is an infection of the lungs due to the aspiration of sucking of food particles, fluid, or vomit, into the lungs (*Stedman's* 2000, 1410).

345. **c** Organizations develop a business continuity plan (BCP) to handle an unexpected computer shutdown caused by an intentional or unintentional event or during a natural disaster (Johns 2011, 993).

346. **c** The basic responsibilities of the quality management department include helping departments or groups of departments with similar issues to identify potential quality problems, assisting determination of the best methods for studying potential problems (for example, survey, chart review, or interview with staff), and participating in regular meetings across the organization, as appropriate, and training organization members on quality and performance improvement methodology, tools, and techniques (Johns 2011, 639).

347. **a** In hospitals and other large healthcare organizations, the board of directors has ultimate responsibility for ensuring the quality of the medical care provided in the organization. In addition, the board is responsible for the organization's fiscal (financial) stability (Johns 2011, 639).

348. **b** Infection control is a system for the prevention of communicable diseases that concentrates on protecting healthcare workers and patients against exposure to disease causing organisms and promotes compliance with applicable legal requirements through early identification of potential sources of contamination and implementation of policies and procedures that limit the spread of disease (Johns 2011, 654, 1141).

349. **c** Risk management programs have three functions: risk identification and analysis, loss prevention and reduction, and claims management (Johns 2011, 653).

350. **c** When doing external benchmarking, the other organizations need not be in the same region of the country, but they should be comparable in terms of patient mix and size. The data from the two hospitals are not comparable because Hospital A discharges more patients than Hospital B. In addition, data on the comparability of severity of illness between the two hospitals is lacking and an informed decision cannot be made (Shaw and Elliott 2012, 44).

351. **a** Dashboards are tools that present metrics from a variety of quality aspects in one concise report. They may present measures of clinical quality (such as infection rates), financial quality, volume, and patient satisfaction. The indicators provide snapshots of all areas of quality to give leaders and communities of interest an overall perspective of the service the organization is providing. Dashboards (like dashboards on a car) are reports of process measures that help leaders know what is currently going on so that they can plan strategically where they want to go next (Johns 2011, 611).

352. **a**   Probably the most important concept in the introductory discussion of quality is that of "measurement." Over the decades of attempting to deal with the issues involved in healthcare quality, healthcare professionals have struggled with where to put the emphasis of their resources. Ultimately, they recognized—with the assistance of the theoretical writings of general industry "quality masters"—that the key to improvement lay in the measurement of the important characteristics of their practice (Johns 2011, 606–611).

353. **c**   Donabedian (1988) contributed significantly to our understanding of measuring quality. He recognized that quality had multiple dimensions that needed to be measured using various types of indicators. He proposed three types of quality indicators: Structure indicators measure the attributes of the setting; process indicators measure the actions by which services are provided; and outcome indicators measure the actual results of care for patients and populations (Johns 2011, 610).

354. **c**   Patients and clients (also known as *customers*) have perceptions and expectations of better or worse (also known as *values*) with respect to the healthcare services (also known as the *product*) that they receive from the healthcare system in all its complexity (also known as the *processes*). The results of their use of the products and processes are known as *outcomes*. The level at which healthcare products and processes and outcomes meet the values of its customers when measured fairly scientifically is the basic definition of *quality* in the United States today (Johns 2011, 604).

355. **b**   Change management is the formal process of introducing change, getting it adopted, and diffusing it throughout the organization (Johns 2011, 1073, 1116).

356. **c**   Blue Cross Blue Shield and commercial health plans have been playing an increasingly important role in providing incentives, such as pay for performance (P4P) or pay for quality (P4Q), where EHRs would be used to support data collection and the reporting of clinical outcomes. Those with better outcomes could receive additional reimbursement or be eligible for grants or other subsidies to support further HIT efforts (Johns 2011, 154).

357. **d**   The key feature of performance improvement as implemented in today's healthcare organizations is that it is a continuous cycle of measurement, analysis, monitoring, planning, designing, and evaluating (Johns 2011, 607).

358. **a**   Brainstorming is highly effective for identifying a number of potential processes that may benefit from improvement efforts and for generating solutions to specific problems. It helps people to begin thinking in new ways and gets them involved in the process. It is an excellent method for facilitating open communication (Johns 2011, 628–629).

359. **a**   Performance management is an ongoing challenge and performance reviews should be conducted as part of performance management to encourage good performance. Information about performance should be collected regularly and shared with the employee, whether the job is coding records or directing a department. Good performance results should be shared to encourage and reward ongoing success (Johns 2011, 1044–1045).

360. **a**   Flow charts help all the team members understand the process in the same way The work involved in developing the flow chart allows the team to thoroughly understand every step in the process as well as the sequence of steps. The flow chart provides a visual picture of each decision point and each event that must be completed. It readily points out places where there are redundancy and complex and problematic areas (Johns 2011, 626–627).

361. **a**   A Pareto chart looks very much like a bar chart except that the highest-ranking item is listed first, followed by the second highest, down to the lowest-ranked item. Its purpose is to display how the team ranked the problems and to allow the team to focus on those problems that may have the biggest potential for improving the process. According to the Pareto Principle, 20% of a problem's sources are responsible for 80% of its actual effects. By concentrating on the "vital few" sources, the team can eliminate a large number of undesirable results (Johns 2011, 632).

362. **a**   Change management is the formal process of introducing change, getting it adopted, and diffusing it throughout the organization. This includes clearing the air and answering questions to reduce fear of, and resistance to, change (Johns 2011, 1073).

363. **b**   Performance improvement is based on several fundamental principles, including: the structure of a system determines its performance, all systems demonstrate variation, improvements rely on the collection and analysis of data that increase knowledge, PI requires the commitment and support of top administration, PI works best when leaders and employees know and share the organization's mission, vision and values, PI efforts take time and require a big investment in people; excellent teamwork is essential; communication must be open, honest, and multidirectional, and success must be celebrated to encourage more success (Johns 2011, 613).

364. **b**   Identifying the problem would be the first step in any decision-making process. A decision cannot be made without first determining what the problem is (Johns 2011, 1071).

365. **b**   Review of the pie chart shows that the emergency department has had significant patient growth over the five-year period. By using this patient profile data for performance improvement the hospital should examine capacity changes for this department (Shaw and Elliott 2012, 60).

366. **a**   The first step in benchmarking is to determine the performance measure to be studied and what is to be accomplished. Once a benchmark for a performance measure is determined, analyzing data collection results becomes more meaningful (Shaw and Elliott 2012, 7).

367. **c**   Quantitative analysis is used by health information management technicians as a method to detect whether elements of the patient's health record are missing, or not complete (Sayles and Trawick 2010, 75–76).

368. **c**   The medical staff department is particularly interested in the ICD-9-CM codes associated with each physician. Because diagnostic codes can identify untoward events that occur during hospitalization, the quality of a physician's services can be identified through reports called physician reappointment summaries. These summaries outline the number of cases by diagnosis and procedure type, LOS, and infection and mortality statistics. At reappointment to a facility's medical staff, code-based reports are required. The medical staff department accumulates these reports and works with the elected or appointed medical staff leadership to ensure that a thorough analysis of each physician's activities takes place before he or she is reappointed to the staff (Schraffenberger and Kuehn 2011, 443).

369. **d**   Data comprehensiveness means that all the required data elements are included in the health record. In essence, comprehensiveness means that the record is complete. In both paper-based and computer-based systems, having a complete health record is critical to the organization's ability to provide excellent patient care and to meet all regulatory, legal, and reimbursement requirements (Johns 2011, 46–47).

370. **b**   The sixth scope of work for QIO shifted from the quality focus of the early 1990s to a payment error prevention role and introduced the Payment Error Prevention Program (Casto and Layman 2011, 35, 37).

371. **c** Family practice has the largest variance with the potential for the most savings (Shaw and Elliott 2012, 63-65).

372. **a** Individual audit results by coder may identify that certain coders are ready to be cross trained in another category of coding. Regardless of the corrective actions taken, the results should become part of each employee's performance evaluation (Schraffenberger and Kuehn 2011, 320).

373. **b** Reading this graph, the full-time coder productivity is higher than part-time coder productivity. The cause for this difference must be identified before any solution can be developed to increase the productivity of the part-time coders (Johns 2011, 534, 1063–1065).

374. **a** In 1918, the hospital standardization movement was inaugurated by the American College of Surgeons (ACS). The purpose of the Hospital Standardization Program was to raise the standards of surgery by establishing minimum quality standards for hospitals. The ACS realized that one of the most important items in the care of any patient was a complete and accurate report of the care and treatment provided during hospitalization (Johns 2011, 6).

375. **a** A performance measure is a tool that allows an organization to compare their performance in comparison to a specific process or outcome. Performance measures include process measures and outcome measures (Shaw and Elliott 2012, 16–17).

376. **b** When an organization compares its current performance to its own internal historical data, or uses data from similar external organizations across the country, it helps establish a benchmark, also known as a standard of performance or best practice, for a particular process or outcome (Shaw and Elliott 2012, 7).

377. **c** Performance measurement in healthcare provides an indication of an organization's performance in relation to a specified process or outcome. Healthcare performance improvement philosophies most often focus on measuring performance in systems, processes and outcomes (Shaw and Elliott 2012, 14).

378. **a** Determining the quickest solution is not a step in the quality improvement decision-making process. Understanding the problem and working through a process to determine the best solution takes time and is not done quickly (Johns 2011, 1071–1073).

379. **c** The principal process by which organizations optimize the continuum of care for their patients is called case management. Case managers review the condition of patients to identify each patient's care needs and to integrate patient data with the patient's course of treatment (Shaw and Elliott 2012, 112).

380. **a** Preadmission care planning is initiated when the patient's physician contacts a healthcare organization to schedule an episode of care service. The case manager reviews the patient's projected needs with the physician. Admission criteria are established based on a suggested diagnosis (Shaw and Elliott 2012, 113).

381. **b** The National Patient Safety Goals (NPSGs) have effectively mandated all healthcare organizations examine care processes that have a potential for error and can cause injury to patients. The NPSGs include identifying patients correctly, improving staff communication, using medicines safely, preventing infection, checking patient medicines, preventing patients from falling, preventing bed sores, and identifying patient safety risks (Shaw and Elliott 2012, 138–140).

382. **b** Performance measurement in healthcare provides an indication of an organization's performance in relation to a specified process or outcome. Healthcare performance improvement philosophies most often focus on measuring performance in systems, processes and outcomes. Processes are the interrelated activities in healthcare organizations that promote effective and safe patient outcomes across services and disciplines within an integrated environment (Shaw and Elliott 2012, 14).

383. **a** An indicator, or criterion, is a performance measure that enables healthcare organizations to monitor a process to determine whether it is meeting process requirements. The criteria may be established and implemented internally, externally, or generically (Shaw and Elliott 2012, 118–119).

384. **a** Credentials are the recognition by healthcare organizations of previous professional practice responsibilities and experiences commonly accorded to licensed independent practitioners and are usually conferred by a national professional organization dedicated to a specific area of healthcare practice (Shaw and Elliott 2012, 284).

385. **d** The level of which healthcare products, processes, and outcomes meets the value of its' customers when measured fairly scientifically is the basic definition of quality (Johns, 2011, 604).

386. **c** A governing body or board of trustees has ultimate legal responsibility for the quality of care rendered in a healthcare organization. Once the bylaws are have been established, however, ultimate responsibility for the quality of documentation is delegated to individual providers who create and authenticate entries in the health record (Brodnik et al. 2012, 171).

387. **c** Medical necessity and utilization review are often reviewed for rehabilitative therapies, inpatient admissions, and mental health and dependency care as well as other conditions. Well baby checks would not be typically reviewed for medical necessity and utilization (Casto and Layman 2011, 99–100).

388. **c** The formulary is composed of medications used for commonly occurring conditions or diagnoses treated in the healthcare organization. Organizations accredited by the Joint Commission are required to maintain a formulary and document that they review it at least annually for a medication's continued safety and efficacy (Shaw and Elliott 2012, 212).

389. **a** Strategic planning is concerned primarily with how the organization will respond to changes in its external environment in the foreseeable future. A step in strategic planning is conducting an environmental assessment. An environmental assessment is a collection of information about changes that have occurred in the organization's internal and external environment since the previous year (Johns 2011, 1053).

390. **d** When a facility evaluates a provider for privileges, it must query the National Practitioner Data Bank for adverse actions taken against providers. Information in the database includes credentialing information, disciplinary actions, medical malpractice settlements or judgments, adverse peer review decisions, professional society memberships. Information regarding personal bankruptcy is not found in the database (Brodnik et al. 2012, 469).

391. **d** The Joint Commission's current quality improvement activities for health record documentation include core performance measures. Seizure disorder is not one of the core measures (Brodnik et al. 2012, 413).

392. **a** Healthcare Effectiveness Data and Information Set (HEDIS) is overseen by the National Committee for Quality Assurance. HEDIS is a standardized set of performance measures designed to allow purchasers to compare the performance of managed-care plans (Sayles and Trawick 2010, 73).

393. **b** When a patient is admitted to the hospital, a case manager will review all the information that has been gathered by the clinicians assigned to the case to confirm that the patient meets the admission criteria for an admitting diagnosis. The case manager will confirm that the patient requires services that can be performed in the facility (Shaw and Elliott 2012, 113).

394. **a** Performance measurement in healthcare provides an indication of an organization's performance in relation to a specified process or outcome. Healthcare performance improvement philosophies most often focus on measuring performance in systems, processes and outcomes. Outcomes are the results of care, treatment, and services in terms of the patient's expectations, needs, and quality of life, which may be positive and appropriate or negative and diminishing (Shaw and Elliott 2012, 14).

395. **a** For a healthcare organization to define optimal care, it must first establish standards of care. Standards of care are an established set of clinical decisions and actions taken by clinicians and other representatives of healthcare organizations in accordance with state and federal laws, regulations, and guidelines; the codes of ethics published by professional associations or societies; the criteria for accreditation published by accreditation agencies; or the usual and common practice of similar clinicians or organizations in a geographical region (Shaw and Elliott 2012, 138).

396. **b** Comparing an organization's performance to the performance of other organizations that provide the same types of service is known as benchmarking. Internal benchmarking is also important to establish a baseline for the organization to find ways to improve effectiveness (Shaw and Elliott 2012, 44).

397. **b** Title IV of Pub. L. 99-660, the Health Care Quality Improvement Act of 1986, created the National Practitioner Data Bank (NPDB). The NPDB is an information clearinghouse created by Congress to improve healthcare quality and reduce healthcare fraud and abuse (Brodnik et al. 2012, 469).

398. **d** The Joint Commission has core measure criteria sets for heart failure, acute myocardial infarction, and pneumonia. Diabetes mellitus is not included as a core measure (Shaw and Elliott 2012, 152).

399. **c** The supervisor should check the new employee's work periodically to ensure the employee understands the training and the work is error free (Johns 2011 1041–1042).

400. **c** The data on the graph show there is a net reduction in overall expenses on a monthly basis for the e-WebCoding system. Learning to use data analysis tools and data aggregation techniques is important for improvement decisions. Making decisions based on actual experience and aggregate data is much better than making decisions on intuition or gut feelings (Shaw and Elliott 2012, 67).

401. **b** The organization as a whole may have an operational plan and each department within the organization creates an annual plan that states its goals and objectives. Operational plans are normally tied to budget planning because of the resources usually required to meet them. Making up the weekly work schedule would be part of operational planning (Johns 2011, 1055, 1062).

402. **a**   Several tools may be used to plan and manage staff resources. For example, position descriptions outline the work and qualifications required by the job. Performance standards establish expectations for how well the job will be done and how much work will be accomplished (Johns 2011, 1060).

403. **c**   Productivity standards need to be set to achieve optimal output. Using work imaging the supervisor could get a snapshot of the current process and then could use that data along with benchmarking data to set productivity standards for the ROI staff (Schraffenberger and Kuehn 2011, 276–279).

404. **a**   Quantitative analysis is used by health information management technicians as a method to detect whether elements of the patient's health record are missing (Sayles and Trawick 2010, 75–76).

405. **b**   Qualitative analysis is a detailed review of a patient's health record for the quality of the documentation contained therein (Sayles and Trawick 2010, 76).

406. **b**   The health record is considered legal documentation of the healthcare services provided to patients. Attorneys for healthcare organizations use it as a tool to protect the legal interests of the facility and its patient care providers (Johns 2011, 38).

407. **a**   An outsourced transcription company and vendor would be business associates of a covered entity (CE). Although business associates are not directly regulated by the Privacy Rule, they do come under the Privacy Rule's requirements by virtue of their association with one or more CEs. A business associate is a person or organization other than a member of a CE's workforce that performs functions or activities on behalf of or affecting a CE that involve the use or disclosure of individually identifiable health information (45 CFR 160.103(1); Brodnik et al. 2012, 220).

408. **d**   With the passage of the Privacy Rule, a minimum amount of protection (that is, a floor) was achieved uniformly across all the states through the establishment of a consistent set of standards that affected providers, healthcare clearinghouses, and health plans (Brodnik et al. 2012, 218).

409. **d**   Competent adults have a general right to consent to or refuse medical treatment. In general, a competent adult has the right to request, receive, examine, copy, and authorize disclosure of the patient's healthcare information (Brodnik et al. 2012, 333).

410. **c**   To meet the individually identifiable element of PHI, information must meet all three portions of a three-part test: it must either identify the person or provide a reasonable basis to believe the person could be identified from the information given; it must relate to one's past, present, or future physical or mental health condition, the provision of health care, or payment for the provision of healthcare; and it must be held or transmitted by a covered entity or it business associate (Brodnik et al. 2012, 221–222).

411. **c**   One of the most fundamental terms in the Privacy Rule is PHI, defined by the rule as "individually identifiable health information that is transmitted by electronic media, maintained in electronic media, or transmitted or maintained in any other form or medium" (45 CFR 160.103). To meet the individually identifiable element of PHI, information must meet all three portions of a three-part test. 1.) It must either identify the person or provide a reasonable basis to believe the person could be identified from the information given. 2.) It must relate to one's past, present, or future physical or mental health condition; the provision of healthcare; or payment for the provision of healthcare. 3.) It must be held or transmitted by a covered entity or its business associate (Brodnik et al. 2012, 221–222).

412. c There are certain circumstances where the minimum necessary requirement does not apply such as to healthcare providers for treatment; to the individual or his personal representative; pursuant to the individual's authorization to the secretary of the HHS for investigations, compliance review, or enforcement; as required by law; or to meet other Privacy Rule compliance requirements (45 CFR 164.502(b)(2); Brodnik et al. 2012, 239–240).

413. c Covered entities (CEs) are responsible for their workforce, which consists not only of employees but also volunteers, student interns, and trainees. Workforce members are not limited to those who receive wages from the CE (45 CFR 160.103; Brodnik et al. 2012, 219).

414. d Vendors who have a presence in a healthcare facility, agency, or organization will often have access to patient information in the course of their work. If the vendor meets the definition of a business associate (that is, it is using or disclosing an individual's PHI on behalf of the healthcare organization), a business associate agreement must be signed. If a vendor is not a business associate, employees of the vendor should sign confidentiality agreements because of their routine contact with and exposure to patient information. In this situation, Ready-Clean is not a business associate (Brodnik et al. 2012, 337).

415. b Although a person or organization may, by definition, be subject to the Privacy Rule by virtue of the type of organization it is, not all information that it holds or comes into contact with is protected by the Privacy Rule. For example, the Privacy Rule has specifically excluded from its scope employment records held by the covered entity in its role as employer (45 CFR 160.103). Under this exclusion, employee physical examination reports contained within personnel files are specifically exempted from this rule (Brodnik et al. 2012, 226).

416. a Another administrative safeguard specification requires that a covered entity implement a security awareness and training program for all members of its workforce. Special protections must be taken to ensure information is not inappropriately released or accessed. These protections include log-in monitoring, password management, and security reminders (Brodnik et al. 2012, 279–280).

417. b Because of cost and space limitations, permanently storing paper and microfilm-based health record documents is not an option for most hospitals. Acceptable destruction methods for paper documents include burning, shredding, pulping, and pulverizing (Odom-Wesley 2009, 69).

418. a A definition of what constitutes a record in each hybrid system must be developed. It is also important to regularly update system descriptions to include the location of all care documents so that patient health information remains readily available to users. A matrix that includes the report/document type, media type, source system, electronic storage start date, and stop printing start date should be maintained by the healthcare organization (Odom-Wesley 2009, 232–233).

419. b The General Rules provide the objective and scope for the HIPAA Security Rule as a whole. They specify that covered entities must develop a security program that includes a range of security safeguards that protect individually identifiable health information maintained or transmitted in electronic form (Johns 2011, 1000).

420. c Administrative safeguards are documented, formal practices to manage data security measures throughout the organization. Basically, they require the facility to establish a security management process. The administrative provisions detail how the security program should be managed from the organization's perspective. Administrative safeguards have nine standards including the development and testing of a contingency plan. This is to ensure that procedures are in place to handle an emergency response in the event of an untoward event such as a power outage (Johns 2011, 1001–1003).

421. **c** Implementation specifications define how standards are to be implemented. Implementation specifications are either "required" or "addressable." Covered entities must implement all implementation specifications that are "required" (Johns 2011, 1000–1001).

422. **d** The Business Record Exception is the rule under which a record is determined to not be hearsay if it was made at or near the time by, or from information transmitted by, a person with knowledge; it was kept in the course of a regularly conducted business activity; and it was the regular practice of that business activity to make the record (Brodnik et al. 2012, 71).

423. **a** Incident reports involving patient care are not created to treat the patient, but rather to provide a basis for investigating the incident. From an evidentiary standpoint, incident reports should not be placed in a patient's health record, nor should the record refer to an incident report (Brodnik et al. 2012, 75–77).

424. **c** Spoliation is a legal concept applicable to both paper and electronic records. When evidence is destroyed that relates to a current or pending civil or criminal proceeding, it is reasonable to infer that the party had a consciousness of guilt or another motive to avoid the evidence (Brodnik et al. 2012, 63–64).

425. **a** Even if evidence appears to be relevant, it must also be authenticated. As with health records, the evidence itself must be shown to have a baseline authenticity or trustworthiness (Brodnik et al. 2012, 67).

426. **b** A court order is a document issued by a judge that compels a certain action, such as testimony or the production of documents such as health records. If a document requesting the production of health records is determined to be a court order, it must be complied with regardless of the presence or absence of patient authorization (Brodnik et al. 2012, 37).

427. **b** Once the validity of the subpoena *duces tecum* has been verified, including the patient's authorization to release the requested records, appropriate measures must be taken to prior to disclosure to ensure the completeness and integrity of the health record. The following steps should be taken: examine the health record for completeness and legibility; ensure the patient's name is present on every page; examine the record to determine if there is a basis for possible negligence action against the provider (and review with legal counsel, if necessary); number the pages; photocopy the record and attempt to submit it in lieu of the original by authenticating the record as an exact replica, etc. Removing pages with detrimental information should never be done (Brodnik et al. 2012, 40–41).

428. **c** Expressed consent is a consent that is either spoken or written. Although courts recognize both spoken and written consent, spoken consent is more difficult to prove (Johns 2011, 71–72).

429. **b** The Privacy Rule introduced the standard that individuals should be informed how covered entities use or disclose PHI. Section 164.520 requires that, except for certain variations or exceptions for health plans and correctional facilities, an individual has the right to a notice explaining how his or her PHI will be used and disclosed. This is the notice of privacy practices (Johns 2011, 836–837).

430. **b** The US Constitution defines and lays out the powers of the three branches of the federal government. The legislative branch (the House of Representatives and the Senate) creates statutory laws (statutes). Examples include Medicare and HIPAA (Johns 2011, 806).

431. **d**   The concept of security is related to privacy and confidentiality. Security describes the physical and electronic protection of health information (Brodnik et al. 2012, 6–7).

432. **d**   The custodian of health records is the individual who has been designated as having responsibility for the care, custody, control, and proper safekeeping and disclosure of health records for such persons or institutions that prepare and maintain records of healthcare (Brodnik et al. 2012, 7).

433. **b**   Ownership of the health record has traditionally been granted to the provider who generates the record (Brodnik et al. 2012, 7).

434. **d**   The process of releasing health record documentation originally created by a different provider is called redisclosure. Federal and state regulations provide specific redisclosure guidelines; however, when in doubt, follow the same principles as the release and disclosure guidelines for other types of health record information (Odom-Wesley 2009, 67).

435. **c**   Healthcare providers with a direct treatment relationship with an individual must provide the notice of privacy practices no later than the date of the first service delivery (for example, first visit to a physician's office, first admission to a hospital, or first encounter at a clinic), including service delivered electronically. Notices must be available at the site where the individual is treated and must be posted in a prominent place where patients can reasonably be expected to read it. If the facility has a website with information on the covered entity's services or benefits, the notice of privacy practices must be prominently posted to it (Johns 2011, 836–838).

436. **c**   A subpoena *duces tecum* means to bring documents and other records with oneself. Such subpoenas may direct the HIT to bring originals or copies of health records, laboratory reports, x-rays, or other records to a deposition or to court. Each state has different rules governing the production of health records in litigation. Often, the component state HIM association of AHIMA has a legal handbook that outlines the various conditions and how HITs should respond to a subpoena (Johns 2011, 809).

437. **c**   A covered entity must act on an individual's request for review of PHI no later than thirty days after the request is made, extending the response period by no more than thirty additional days if it gave the individual a written statement within the thirty-day time period explaining the reasons for the delay and the date by which the covered entity will complete its action on the request. The covered entity may extend the time for action on a request for access only once (Johns 2011, 829, 831).

438. **a**   The Privacy Rule introduced the standard of minimum necessary to limit the amount of PHI used, disclosed, and requested. This means that healthcare providers and other covered entities must limit uses, disclosures, and requests to only the amount needed to accomplish the intended purpose. For example, for payment purposes, only the minimum amount of information necessary to substantiate a claim for payment should be disclosed (Johns 2011, 822).

439. **c**   Under the Privacy Rule, healthcare providers are not required to obtain patient consent to use or disclose personal identifiable information for treatment, payment, and healthcare operations (Johns 2011, 838).

440. **c**   Privacy is when a patient has the right to maintain control over certain health information (Johns 2011, 755).

441. **b** Confidentiality, as recognized by law and professional codes of ethics, stems from a relationship such as physician and patient, and pertains to the information resulting from that relationship. Privileged communication is a legal concept designed to protect the confidentiality between two parties (Brodnik et al. 2012, 5–6).

442. **b** Agreements between the covered entity and a business associate includes: requires the business associate to make available all of its books and records relating to PHI use and disclosure to the Department of Health and Human Services or its agent; prohibits the business associate from using or disclosing PHI in any way that would violate the HIPAA Privacy Rule; and prohibits the business associate form using or disclosing PHI for any purpose other than that described in the contract with the covered entity; and other agreements. But, it does not allow the business associate to maintain PHI indefinitely (Johns 2011, 824–825).

443. **c** A covered entity must act on an individual's request for review of PHI no later than 30 days after the request is made, extending the response period by no more than 30 additional days if it gave the individual a written statement within the 30 day time period explaining the reasons for the delay and the date by which the covered entity will complete its action on the request. The covered entity may extend the time for action on a request for access only once. If PHI is not maintained or located on-site, the covered entity is given within 60 days of receipt to respond to a request (Johns 2011, 829, 831).

444. **b** The CSO is responsible for developing the security goals and objectives for the covered entity; determining how the goals and objectives will be met; advising administration regarding information security; determining reporting procedures; and conducting adequate risk assessment (Sayles and Trawick 2010, 305).

445. **a** Although business associates are not directly regulated by the Privacy Rule, they do come under the Privacy Rule's requirements by virtue of their association with one or more covered entities. Some examples of business associates are: contract coder, billing companies, consultants, accounting firms, etc. (Brodnik et al. 2012, 220).

446. **c** Hospitals and other healthcare facilities develop health record retention policies to ensure that health records comply with all applicable state and federal regulations, accreditation standards, as well as meet future patient care needs. Most states have established regulations that address how long health records and other healthcare-related documents must be maintained before they can be destroyed (Odom-Wesley 2009, 67).

447. **a** The covered entity may require the individual to make an amendment request in writing and provide a rationale for their amendment request. Such a process must be communicated in advance to the individual (Brodnik 2012, 242).

448. **a** A patient has the opportunity to agree or disagree with being placed in a patient directory. They must be given the opportunity to determine if they want to be placed in the directory or not, but it does not need to be in writing (Johns 2011, 839, 842).

449. **b** PHI stands for protected health information (Johns 2011, 819).

450. **a** AHIMA outlines the requirements for the content of the notice of privacy practices. One requirement is that a description (including at least one example) is to be given of the types of uses and disclosures the covered entity is permitted to make for treatment, payment, and healthcare operations (Johns 2011, 836–837).

451. **a**   The legal health record is record that will be disclosed upon request by third parties. It includes documentation about health services provided and stored on any media (Johns 2011, 815–816).

452. **d**   An individual may revoke an authorization at any time, provided that he or she does so in writing. However, the revocation does not apply when the covered entity has already taken action on the authorization (Brodnik 2012, 238).

453. **c**   Covered entities may disclose PHI to public health entities even if the law does not specifically require the disclosure is for the purpose of preventing or controlling disease; injury; or disability; including, but not limited to, the reporting of disease; injury; vital events such as birth or death; and the conduct of public health surveillance (Brodnik et al. 2012, 395).

454. **a**   Nonmaleficence would require the HIM professional to ensure that the information is not released to someone who does not have authorization to access it and who might harm the patient if access were permitted (for example, a newspaper seeking information about a famous person) (Johns 2011, 752).

455. **c**   Once litigation can be reasonably anticipated, an organization should establish a legal (litigation) hold, and reasonable measure should be taken to identify and preserve all information relevant to the claim. A legal hold (also know as a preservation order) may or may not be issued by a court. Making a copy of the health record and securing the original in a locked location would fulfill the organization's requirement for a legal hold (Odom-Wesley, 2009, 270–271).

456. **b**   Upon being awarded the credential of registered health information technician (RHIT) or registered health information administrator (RHIA) by the American Health Information Management Association (AHIMA), the HIM professional agrees to follow ethical principles and to base all professional actions and decisions on those principles and values. Even if federal or state laws did not require the protection of patient privacy, the HIM professional would be responsible for protecting it according to AHIMA's Code of Ethics (Johns 2011, 757).

457. **c**   The Privacy Rule addresses the issue of personal representatives. Personal representatives are those who are legally authorized to make healthcare decisions on a individual's behalf or to act on behalf of a deceased individual or that individual's estate. Under the Privacy Rule, then, a personal representative must be treated the same as the individual regarding the use and disclosure of the individual's PHI. In this instance, the fact that the sister is listed in the health record as the caregiver does not make her legally authorized as a personal representative under the Privacy Rule. Her request should be refused (Brodnik et al. 2012, 224).

458. **c**   The HIPAA Privacy Rule concept of "minimum necessary" does not apply to disclosures made for treatment purposes. However, the covered entity must define, within the organization, what information physicians need as part of their treatment role (Thomason and Dennis 2008, 3).

459. **d**   A person's right to privacy is the right to be left alone and protected against physical or psychological invasion. It includes freedom from intrusion into one's private affairs to include their healthcare diagnoses (Brodnik et. al. 2012, 5).

460. **b**   When entries are made in the health record regarding a patient who is particularly hostile or irritable, general documentation principles apply, such as charting objective facts and avoiding the use of personal opinions, particularly those that are critical of the patient. The degree to which these general principles apply is heightened because a disagreeable patient may cause a provider to use more expressive and inappropriate language. Further, a hostile patient may be more likely to file legal action in the future if the hostility is a personal attribute and not simply a manifestation of his or her medical condition (Brodnik et al. 2012, 173).

461. **a**   The health record may be valuable evidence in a legal proceeding. To be admissible, the court must be confident that the record is: complete, accurate, and timely (recorded at the time the event occurred); was documented in the normal course of business; and was made by healthcare providers who have knowledge of the "acts, events, conditions, opinions, or diagnoses appearing in it" (Brodnik et al. 2012,67).

462. **a**   Illegible physician documentation can result in serious harm or injury to a patient. One of the most embarrassing and damning ploys by a plaintiff's attorney can use during a trial for malpractice is to show that a physician cannot understand or read his or her own health record entries. Complete and accurate health record documentation is the foundation of effective risk management (Johns 2011, 658–660).

463. **c**   The OPPS is the Medicare prospective payment system used for hospital-based outpatient services and procedures that is predicated on the assignment of ambulatory payment classifications. The radiology examinations would be reimbursed under this system (Johns 2011, 330).

464. **b**   As a result of the disparity in documentation practices by providers, querying has become a common communication and educational method to advocate proper documentation practices. Queries can be made in situations when there is clinical evidence for a higher degree of specificity or severity (Schraffenberger and Kuehn 2011, 42).

465. **b**   Medicaid charges are larger than the charges to commercial insurance and TRICARE, however, the facility receives a smaller payment from Medicaid. There is an adjustment of 36%, meaning that the facility had to adjust their charges 36% from the actual amount billed and the amount they receive in payment (Johns 2011, 355–356).

466. **d**   Revenue cycle management is the supervision of all administrative and clinical functions that contribute to the capture, management, and collection of patient service revenue (Casto and Layman 2011, 249).

467. **c**   Accounts Receivable manages the amounts owed to a facility by customers who received services but whose payments will be made at a later date by the patients or their third-party payers. Once the claim is submitted to third-party payer for reimbursement, the Accounts Receivable clock begins to tick (Casto and Layman 2011, 253).

468. **a**   Dollars in accounts receivable is the amount of money owed a healthcare facility after the claim has been submitted (Casto and Layman 2011, 253).

469. **d**   The last component of the revenue cycle is reconciliation and collections. The healthcare facility uses the EOB, MSN, and RA to reconcile accounts. These are monitored in the claims reconciliation and collections area of the revenue cycle (Casto and Layman 2011, 254).

470. **b**   Most CFOs and patient account directors consider coding to be the HIM departments most significant function (Schraffenberger and Kuehn 2011, 468).

471. **b**   When all third-party payments have been received and contractual allowances have been written off, the remaining balance is categorized as the patient responsibility. Best practice is to have the patient responsibility amount be less than 15% of the total balance (Schraffenberger and Kuehn 2011, 460).

472. **a**   At this time, several types of hospitals are excluded from Medicare acute inpatient prospective payment system (PPS) because the PPS diagnosis-related groups do not accurately account for the resource costs for the types of patients treated in those facilities. The following facilities are still paid on the basis of reasonable cost: psychiatric and rehabilitation hospitals, long-term care hospitals, children's hospitals, cancer hospitals, and critical access hospitals (Johns 2011, 322).

473. **c**   To accept assignment means the provider or supplier accepts, as payment in full, the allowed charge. The provider or supplier is prohibited from balance billing, which means the patient cannot be held responsible for charges in excess of the Medicare fee schedule (Johns 2011, 350).

474. **d**   The outpatient prospective payment system (OPPS) was first implemented for services furnished on or after August 1, 2000. Under the OPPS, the federal government pays for hospital outpatient services on a rate-per-service basis that varies according to the ambulatory payment classification (APC) group to which the service is assigned. The Healthcare Common Procedural Coding System (HCPCS) identifies and groups the services within each APC group. Services included under APCs follow: surgical procedures, radiology, clinical visits, ER visits, partial hospitalization services for the mentally ill, chemotherapy, preventative services and screening exams, dialysis for other than ESRD, vaccines, splints, casts, antigens, and certain implantable items (Johns 2011, 329–330).

475. **b**   The outpatient prospective payment system (OPPS) was first implemented for services furnished on or after August 1, 2000. Under the OPPS, the federal government pays for hospital outpatient services on a rate-per-service basis that varies according to the ambulatory payment classification (APC) group to which the service is assigned. The Healthcare Common Procedural Coding System (HCPCS) identifies and groups the services within each APC group. Services included under APCs follow: surgical procedures, radiology, clinical visits, ER visits, partial hospitalization services for the mentally ill, chemotherapy, preventative services and screening exams, dialysis for other than ESRD, vaccines, splints, casts, antigens, and certain implantable items (Johns 2011, 329–330).

476. **a**   The Medicare fee schedule is prepared each year (Johns 2011, 326).

477. **a**   Physicians submit claims via the electronic format (screen 837P), which takes the place of the CMS-1500 billing form (Johns 2011, 343).

478. **b**   Medicare participation means that the provider or supplier agrees to accept assignment for all covered services provided to Medicare patients. To accept assignment means the provider or supplier accepts, as payment in full, the allowed charge (from the fee schedule). The provider or supplier is prohibited from balance billing, which means the patient cannot be held responsible for charges in excess of the Medicare fee schedule (Johns 2011, 350).

479. **a**   In many instances, patients have more than one insurance policy and the determination of which policy is primary and which is secondary is necessary so that there is no duplication in payment of benefits. This process is called the coordination of benefits (COB) or the coordination of benefits transaction. The monies collected from third-party payers cannot be greater than the amount of the provider's charges (Johns 2011, 343).

480. **d**   Facilities may design the CDI program based on several different models. Improvement work can be done with retrospective record review and queries, with concurrent record review and queries, or with concurrent coding. Staffing models may include the involvement of the CDS discussed previously or could be done by enhancing the role of the utilization review staff or case managers, or a combination of these models. Retrospective review of all query opportunities for the year would help to validate the effectiveness of the new program (Schraffenberger and Kuehn 2011, 363).

481. **b**   The Medicare Provider Analysis and Review (MEDPAR) file is made up of acute care hospital and skilled nursing facility (SNF) claims data for all Medicare claims. The MEDPAR file is frequently used for research on topics such as charges for particular types of care and DRGs. The limitation of the MEDPAR data for research purposes is that the file contains only Medicare patients (Johns 2011, 498).

482. **b**   Part of the Health Insurance Portability and Accountability Act of 1996 (HIPAA) mandated the collection of information on healthcare fraud and abuse because there was no central place to obtain this information. As a result, the national Healthcare Integrity and Protection Data Bank (HIPDB) was developed (Johns 2011, 499).

483. **b**   TRICARE, formerly known as Civilian Health and Medical Program of the Uniformed Services (CHAMPUS), is a healthcare program for active duty service members, National Guard and Reserve members, retirees, their families, survivors and certain former spouses (Johns 2011, 305).

484. **a**   Inpatient hospital care is limited to 90 days in each benefit period. When a beneficiary exhausts the 90 days, a non-renewable lifetime reserve of 60 days of additional care can be used. In this case the beneficiary has used 36 of the 60 days, which leaves 24 remaining days (Johns 2011, 294–295).

485. **a** $85 \times 0.20 = $17 co-insurance. A $15 copay is lower than the 20% ($17) co-insurance (Johns 2011, 288).

486. **d**   SNF care is covered when a patient requires skilled nursing or rehabilitation services occurring within 30 days of a three-day-long or longer acute hospitalization and is certified as medically necessary. The number of SNF days provided under Medicare is limited to 100 days per benefit period. Medicare fully covers the first 20 days in a benefit period. For days 21 through 100, a copayment ($144.50 per day in 2012) is required. Medicare benefits expire after the first 100 days of SNF care during a benefit period (Johns 2011, 295).

487. **a**   Medicare Part A or B does not usually cover the following services: long-term nursing care, custodial care, dentures and dental care, eyeglasses, and hearing aids (Johns 2011, 294–297).

488. **d**   TRICARE, formerly known as Civilian Health and Medical Program of the Uniformed Services (CHAMPUS), is a healthcare program for active-duty service members, National Guard, and Reserve members, retirees, their families, survivors, and certain former spouses (Johns 2011, 305).

489. **c**   Title XIX of the Social Security Act enacted Medicaid in 1965. State governments work with the federal Medicaid program to provide healthcare coverage to low-income individuals and families. The Medicaid program pays for medical assistance provided to individuals and families with low incomes and limited financial resources (Johns 2011, 301).

490. **c**   For those enrolled in both programs, any services covered by Medicare are paid for by the Medicare program before any payments are made by the Medicaid program because Medicaid is always the payer of last resort (Johns 2011, 303).

491. **a**   PPOs represent contractual agreements between healthcare providers and a self-insured employer or a health insurance carrier. Beneficiaries of PPOs select providers such as physicians or hospitals from a list of participating providers who have agreed to furnish healthcare services to the covered population (Johns 2011, 311).

492. **b**   In a prospective payment system (PPS), the exact amount of the payment is determined before the service is delivered (Johns 2011, 315, 690–691).

493. **a** Global payment methodology is sometimes applied to radiological and similar types of procedures that involve professional and technical components. Global payments are lump-sum payments distributed among the physicians who performed the procedure or interpreted its results and the healthcare facility that provided the equipment, supplies, and technical support required (Johns 2011, 318).

494. **b** The claims processing area uses an internal auditing system to ensure claims are error free. Once all data have been posted to a patient's account, the claim can be reviewed for accuracy and completeness. Many facilities have internal auditing systems known as scrubbers. The auditing system runs each claim through a set of edits specifically designed for the third-party payer; identifying data that has failed edits and flags the claim for correction (Casto and Layman 2011, 252).

495. **a** Medicare claims for Part A services and hospital based Medicare Part B services are submitted to a designated Medicare administrative contractor (MAC). MACs are replacing the claims payment contractors known as fiscal intermediaries (Casto and Layman 2011, 254).

496. **a** Revenue cycle management involves different processes and people, all working to make sure that the healthcare facility is properly reimbursed for the services provided. Effectively managing the revenue cycle is paramount to improving the revenues received by the facility. Transposition of digits in the patient's social security number, date of birth, or policy number would all result in a delay in reimbursement and negatively impact an organizations revenue cycle management(Johns 2011, 355).

497. **b** Claims processing activities include the capture of all billable services, claim generation, and claim correction. Charge capture is a vital component of the revenue cycle (Casto and Layman 2011, 250).

498. **d** Individual states must meet broad national guidelines established by federal statutes, regulations, and policies to qualify for federal matching grants under the Medicaid program. Individual state medical assistance agencies, however, establish the Medicaid eligibility standards for residents of their states. The states also determine the type, amount, duration, and scope of covered services; calculate the rate of payment for covered services; and administer local programs. Medicaid policies on eligibility, services, and payment are complex and vary considerably among states. Therefore, an individual who is eligible for Medicaid in one state may not be eligible in another (Johns 2011, 301).

499. **c** SCHIP (sometimes referred to as the Children's Health Insurance Program, or CHIP) allows states to expand existing insurance programs to cover children up to age 19. It provides additional federal funds to states so that Medicaid eligibility can be expanded to include a greater number of children (Johns 2011, 304).

500. **a** The principal purpose of the CDM is to allow the healthcare facility to efficiently and accurately charge repetitive services and routine supplies to the patient's bill. Through the process of order entry, services located in the CDM are "charges" to the patient's account as they are rendered to the patient (Schraffenberger and Kuehn 2011, 223).

501. **c** Late charges are any charges that have not been posted to the account number within the healthcare facility's established bill hold time period. Best practice is four days from the date of service/discharge. For the provider to be paid for these charges, an adjusted claim must be sent to Medicare (Schraffenberger and Kuehn 2011, 460).

502. **c**   When patients have more than one insurance policy, the determination of which policy is primary and which is secondary is necessary so there is not duplication in payment of benefits. This process is called the coordination of benefits (COB) or the coordination of benefits transaction. The monies collected from third-party payers cannot be greater than the amount of the provider's charges (Johns 2011, 343).

503. **b**   The IHS is an agency within the HHS. It is responsible for providing healthcare services to American Indians and Alaska natives. The American Indians and Alaska natives served by the IHS receive preventive healthcare services, primary medical services (hospital and ambulatory care), community health services, substance abuse treatment services, and rehabilitative services. Secondary medical care, highly specialized medical services, and other rehabilitative care are provided by IHS staff or by private healthcare professionals working under contract with the HIS (Johns 2011, 306).

504. **d**   Most employees are eligible for some type of workers' compensation insurance. Workers' compensation programs cover healthcare costs and lost income associated with work-related injuries and illnesses (Johns 2011, 306).

505. **a**   Medicare Part A coverage is measured in "benefit periods." In each benefit period there are limits to the number of days Medicare will pay for inpatient care. Inpatient hospital care is usually limited to 90 days during each benefit period. A benefit period begins on the day of admission and ends when the beneficiary has been out of the hospital for 60 days in a row, including the day of discharge. There is no limit to the number of benefit periods (Johns 2011, 295).

506. **c**   In this example, DNFB met the benchmark in January, February, and June, which is 3/6 or 50% of the time (Schraffenber and Kuehn 2011, 461).

507. **a**   When patients have more than one insurance policy, a determination of which policy is primary and which is secondary is necessary so there is not duplication in payment of benefits. This process is called the coordination of benefits (COB) or the coordination of benefits transaction. The monies collected from third-party payers cannot be greater than the amount of the provider's charges. If an overpayment occurs, these monies should be returned to correct payer or patient who over paid the claim (Johns 2011, 343).

508. **c**   The charge code (also known as the item code) is the numerical identification of the service or supply. Each line item has a hospital-specific, unique number (Schraffenberger and Kuehn 2011, 225).

509. **d**   Each service or supply item in the CDM is commonly referred to as a line item. Each line item typically has at a minimum the following seven elements: charge code, item description, general ledger (G/L) key, revenue code, CPT/HCPCS code, charge, and activity date (Schraffenberger and Kuehn 2011, 225).

510. **c**   For Medicare and most other third-party payer reporting, Levels I and II of HCPCS codes are used to report supplies and services for the CDM (Schraffenberger and Kuehn 2011, 226).

511. **b**   Focused selections of coded accounts are necessary for deeper understanding of patterns of error or change in high-risk areas or other areas of specific concern (Schraffenberger and Kuehn 2011, 271).

512. **a**   Lower weighted DRGs could have fewer CCs and MCCs, which may be the result of a coder missing secondary diagnoses. A focused audit based on this specific potential problem area could help to identify these cases (Schraffenberger and Kuehn 2011, 314–315).

513. **d** Each of these percentages should be tracked within the first few months of program operation. The target percentage may need adjustment over time as the CDS staff becomes more familiar with their responsibilities and physician documentation improves. These percentages are: record review rate, query rate, query response rate, and query agreement rate (Schraffenberger and Kuehn 2011, 365).

514. **d** The CDS will review the case periodically to check for the physician's response. If no response is given prior to discharge, the information is requested post discharge. If a response is given and the diagnosis changes the MS-DRG, this change is tracked. For longer stays, the CDS will return to the record every 24 to 48 hours to access new documentation (Schraffenberger and Kuehn 2011, 364; Blackford and Whitehouse 2007; Russo 2010).

515. **c** The BBA of 1997 focused on healthcare fraud and abuse issues, especially as they related to penalties. The circumstances under which civil monetary penalties are applied were based on the BBA (Schraffenberger and Kuehn 2011, 373).

516. **b** Diagnostic service provided to a Medicare beneficiary by the admitting hospital, or by an entity wholly owned or wholly operated by the hospital, within three days prior to and including the day of admission are considered to be inpatient services and included in the inpatient payment. The following services are not subject to the three-day payment window rule and are excluded from the inpatient payment: hospice, home health, skilled nursing services, ambulance, or maintenance renal dialysis services with three days of admission (Schraffenberger and Kuehn 2011, 395).

517. **c** Bad debt refers to accounts that show money owed by the patient and that the healthcare facility has defined as uncollectable. When multiple, extensive attempts have been made to collect, but no money has been paid, these charges are written off as bad debt (Schraffenberger and Kuehn 2011, 460).

518. **b** Bill hold is an established time between the date of service and the date the claim is sent to the payer. This time is to allow all charges to be entered and all coding to be completed. The best practice for bill hold is four days from the date of service/discharge (Schraffenberger and Kuehn 2011, 460).

519. **a** Discharged not final billed (DNFB) refers to accounts where the patient has been discharged but the charges have not been processed or billed. The DNFB report is usually "owned" by the HIM department. Because the HIM department codes the health records, any uncoded records, for whatever reason, become the responsibility of the HIM department. Unfortunately, the reason why an account cannot be coded has little to do with HIM operations. More often, uncoded accounts are the result of untimely documentation, misposted charges, registration or the wrong service area, services provided under an incorrect revenue code, or lost paperwork (Schraffenberger and Kuehn 2011, 461).

520. **d** The Integrated Outpatient Code Editor (IOCE) is a predefined set of edits created by Medicare to check outpatient claims for compliance with the Medicare outpatient prospective payment system (OPPS). The IOCE will review a coded claim for accuracy and send back an edit flag if an error has been detected in the claim. Most organizations run all their claims through the IOCE prior to sending out to any payer to look for errors, correct them, and then send out a clean claim. A portion of the NCCI edits are embedded in the IOCE edits (Schraffenberger and Kuehn 2011, 465).

38/58 = 66%

Exam 1

1. **d** The Uniform Hospital Discharge Data Set (UHDDS) characteristics include patient-specific date items on every inpatient, collected by all short-term general hospitals in the United States, and incorporated into federal regulations Medicare and Medicaid (Odom-Wesley et al. 2009, 85).

2. **c** The Uniform Ambulatory Care Data Set (UACDS) is used in every facility for outpatient care (Odom-Wesley et al. 2009, 85).

3. **c** Vocabulary standards are a common definition for medical terms to encourage consistent descriptions of an individual's condition in the health record (Johns 2011, 236).

4. **a** Patient care managers are responsible for the overall evaluation of services rendered for their particular area of responsibility. To identify patterns and trends, they take details from individual health records and then put all the information together in one place. On the basis of these combined aggregate data, the managers recommend changes to patient care processes, equipment, and services (Johns 2011, 36–37).

5. **b** The amount of space, volume of records, and record usage or activity must be considered when determining the type of storage system to use. When space is not sufficient to house the number of shelving units needed to hold the records for the period of time required for patient care and other purposes, older health records are purged or removed from the file area. Generally, files that have been inactive for a certain period of time (for example, three years since the patient's last visit) are removed from the active filing area (Johns 2011, 397).

6. **b** The results of the inventory indicate a significant problem and should not be ignored. Before in-service training or memos can be developed the organization's formal position on data dictionaries must be established (Johns 2011, 1026).

7. **b** Careful attention must be given to ensure that data stored in a database have data quality characteristics including accuracy, accessibility, comprehensiveness, consistency, currency, definition, granularity, and timeliness (Johns 2011, 908).

8. **b** Data content standards allow organizations to collect data once and use it many times in many ways. It also assists in data storage and mining as well as sharing data with external organizations for benchmarking. The HIM director should identify data content requirements for all areas of the organization to ensure the data content standards (Sayles and Trawick 2010, 255).

9. **b** Data consistency means that the data are reliable. Reliable data do not change no matter how many times or in how many ways they are stored, processed, or displayed. Data values are consistent when the value of any given data element is the same across applications and systems. Related data items also should be reliable. For example, the clinical history for a male patient would not likely include a hysterectomy as a past surgical procedure (Johns 2011, 47).

10. **a** The consultation report documents the clinical opinion of a physician other than the primary or attending physician. The consultation is requested by the primary or attending physician. The report is based on the consulting physician's examination of the patient and a review of his or her health record (Johns 2011, 62).

11. **a**   The problem-oriented health record is better suited to serve the patient and the end user of the patient information. The key characteristic of this format is an itemized list of the patient's past and present social, psychological, and medical problems. Each problem is indexed with a unique number (Johns 2011, 114).

12. **c**   Medicare has the highest payment percentage (42%) of any of the payers (Johns 2011, 535).

13. **b**   All states have a health department with a division that is required to track and record communicable diseases. When a patient is diagnosed with one of the diseases from the health department's communicable disease list, the facility must notify the state public health department (Shaw and Elliott 2012, 157–159).

14. **c**   Data about patients can be extracted from individual health records and combined as aggregate data. Aggregate data are used to develop information about groups of patients. For example, data about all of the patients who suffered an acute myocardial infarction during a specific time period could be collected in a database. From the aggregate data, it would be possible to identify common characteristics that might predict the course of the disease or provide information about the most effective way to treat it (Johns 2011, 197).

15. **b**   Clinical laboratory reports would need to be reviewed to determine if a PTT test was performed. Medication records would need to be reviewed to determine if heparin was given after the PTT test was performed (Johns 2011, 68–71).

16. **c**   The Medicare Provider Analysis and Review (MEDPAR) file is made up of acute care hospital and skilled nursing facility (SNF) claims data for all Medicare claims. The MEDPAR file is frequently used for research on topics such as charges for particular types of care and DRGs. The limitation of the MEDPAR data for research purposes is that the file contains only Medicare patients (Johns 2011, 498).

17. **d**   The vital signs record is comprised of blood pressure readings, temperature, respiration, and pulse making it the best source to gather the information (Johns 2011, 65).

18. **c**   The median is the midpoint of a frequency distribution. It is the point at which 50% of observations fall above and 50% fall below. If an even number of observations is in the frequency distribution, the median is the midpoint between the two middle observations. It is found by averaging the two middle scores, $(x + y) / 2$. In the following example, the median is 31.5: ($[30 + 33] / 2$) (Johns 2011, 531).

19. **c**   A table is an orderly arrangement of values that groups data into rows and columns. Almost any type of quantitative information can be organized into tables. Tables are useful for demonstrating patterns and other kinds of relationships. They also may serve as the basis for more visual displays of data, such as charts and graphs, where some of the detail may be lost. A table should contain all the information the user needs to understand the data in it. Tables need headings for columns and rows and they need to be specific and understandable (Johns 2011, 535).

20. **b** $[(250 + 30) - 40] + 2 = 242$. The number of inpatient service days for a 24-hour period is equal to the daily inpatient census—that is, one service day for each patient treated (Johns 2011, 548).

21. **a**   The goal of the ORYX initiative is to integrate outcomes and other performance measures into the accreditation process through data collection about specific core measures (Joint Commission 2009). The core measures are based on selected diagnoses/conditions such as diabetes mellitus, the outcomes of which can be improved by standardizing care. They include the minimum number of data elements needed to provide an accurate and reliable measure of performance (Johns 2011, 211–212).

22. **d**   Filing accuracy can be checked by conducting a random audit of the storage area. To conduct a study a section of the permanent file room can be checked for misfiles. Any files found or noted, and a filing accuracy rate can be determined and compared against the established standard. In this scenario, there were 591 instances of accurate filing out of 600 sampled (591 / 600) $\times$ 100 = 98.5% accuracy (Johns 2011, 417).

23. **a**   The unit numbering system is most commonly used in large healthcare facilities. One advantage to this method is that all information, regardless of the number of encounters, can be filed or linked together. Having all the information related to the patient filed in one location facilitates communication among caregivers and improves operational efficiency (Johns 2011, 387–388).

24. **c**   An important characteristic of results retrieval technologies is that the screen layout can be customized to the user's preference. Many EHR systems display a tailored screen based on the user's logon. Thus, when Dr. Jones logs on, his personally preferred screen layout is displayed (Johns 2011, 165).

25. **b**   In healthcare, the authority file is usually the master patient index (MPI). The filing clerk searches the MPI by patient name. When the correct patient is located in the MPI, the clerk uses the health record number to locate the patient's health record folder within the filing system (Johns 2011, 392).

26. **b**   The integrated health record format organizes all the paper forms in strict chronological order and mixes the forms created by different departments (Johns 2011, 50).

27. **b**   Today's electronic media have generally been found to be sufficiently durable, but the bigger issue relates to whether old media can be read using newer hardware with newer software. As a result, organizations now also have to implement a process of managing hardware obsolescence. Many organizations make new copies of their backups periodically to ensure their permanence and reflect changes in software. HIM professionals should take an active role in managing retention of EHRs, just as they do in managing the retention of paper-based records (Johns 2011, 186).

28. **a**   Three rules apply for alphabetical filing: File each record alphabetically by the last name, followed by the first name and middle initial; last names beginning with a prefix or containing an apostrophe are filed in strict alphabetical order; in hyphenated names such as Manasse-O'Brien, the hyphenation is ignored and the record is filed as Manasseobrien (Johns 2011, 392).

29. **d**   Timeliness of the storage and retrieval processes can be monitored. In this situation, each clinic visit represents a patient record that will need to be retrieved (or pulled) and stored (filed back). (500 / 50) + (500 / 40) = 22.5 hours/day (Johns 2011, 418).

⭐ 30. **a** It is asking for the least amount of hours needed to meet the 24-hour turnaround time. The average discharge in a 24-hour period is 120 patients, and the average pages for each patient chart is 200. (120 × 200 = 24,000 pages in a 24-hour period.) Each chart must be prepped, scanned, checked for quality, and indexed. The highest number of pages that can go through all these processes in an hour would be: 500 images in prepping; 2,400 images in scanning; 2,000 images in quality control; and 800 images in indexing.

- 24, 000 / 500 = 48 hours needed for prepping
- 24,000 / 2,400 = 10 hours for scanning
- 24,000 / 2,000 =12 hours for quality control
- 24,000 / 800 = 30 hours for indexing
- 48 + 10 + 12 + 30 = 100 hours, at least, needed each day to meet a 24-hour turnaround time

Workflow is the process, progress, or flow of the work within a system. The system generally begins with the input, the process to complete the task (such as staff and tools), and ends with the desired output. Also included in the process is the rate at which it happens. Understanding the workflow within a department is crucial for the supervisor in managing the departmental resources. To understand and control the workflow, the supervisor can perform a workflow analysis and then design the process to be more effective and efficient (Johns 2011, 1065).

31. **b** The main purpose of DSM-IV-TR is to provide a means to record data on patients treated for substance abuse and mental disorders. DSM is used as a nomenclature that clinicians can reference to enhance their clinical practices and as a language for communicating diagnostic information. Clinicians use DSM to assign a diagnosis (Johns 2011, 262).

32. **a** The database management system is the best option to collect, store, manipulate and retrieve data for this problem. Paper and word-processing documents cannot sort and store the data in a meaningful way for this problem. Spreadsheets should be used for accounting-type functions and not for data storage (Johns 2011, 902).

33. **d** According to the American Hospital Association's Central Office on ICD-9-CM, ICD-9-CM has a number of uses. Some of these uses are conducting epidemiological and clinical research, storing and retrieving data, and reporting and compiling healthcare data to assist in the evaluation of medical care planning for healthcare delivery systems. Collecting data about nursing care is not a use of ICD-9-CM (Johns 2011, 239).

34. **c** Completeness is the degree to which the codes capture all the diagnoses and procedures documented in the health record (Johns 2011, 266).

⭐ 35. **d** The latest version of the Medicare integrated outpatient code editor (IOCE) should be installed to review claims prior to releasing billed data to the Medicare program. IOCE software contains the National Correct Coding Initiative (NCCI) edits for CPT. The NCCI edits were created to evaluate the relationships between CPT codes on the bill and to control improper coding leading to inappropriate payment on the Part B claims. They also identify component codes that were used instead of the appropriate comprehensive code, as well as other types of coding errors (Schraffenberger and Kuehn 2011, 230).

36. **c** The principal diagnosis is governed by the circumstances of admission which in this case is dehydration (Schraffenberger 2012, 66).

⭐ 37. **a** The calculation of payment for services under the Outpatient Prospective Payment System is based on the categorization of outpatient services into APC groups according to CPT/HCPCS code (Johns 2011, 330).

38. **c**   Option "c" is the only procedure code listed (Johns 2011, 244).

39. **d**   Because this patient was seen only in the emergency department, he or she would be classified as an outpatient. Diagnoses documented as "probable," "suspected," "questionable," "rule out," or "working diagnosis" or other similar terms in the outpatient setting indicate uncertainty, and would not be coded as if existing. Rather, code the condition to the highest degree of certainty for that encounter/visit, such as signs, symptoms, abnormal test results, or other reason for the visit. In this case, unspecified chest pain would be coded (Schraffenberger 2012, Appendix I, 81).

40. **a**   Coders should be evaluated at least quarterly with appropriate training needs identified, facilitated, and reassessed over time. Only through this continuous process of evaluation can data quality and integrity be accurately measured and ensured. Accuracy of coding is best determined by a predefined audit process (Schraffenberger and Kuehn 2011, 63).

☆ 41. **c**   Only one code should be used. The code representing the largest tumor should be used. Large bladder tumors are for tumors 5.0 centimeters or larger (Smith 2012, 60).

42. **b**   No mention is made of biopsy, excision of lesion, or occlusion, so following proper steps for coding in CPT, the correct code is 58670 (Kuehn 2012, 27).

43. **b**   In cases of a cesarean delivery, the selection of the principal diagnosis should be the condition established after study that was responsible for the patient's admission. If the patient was admitted with a condition that resulted in the performance of the cesarean procedure, that condition should be selected as the principal diagnosis. If the reason for the admission/encounter was unrelated to the condition resulting in the cesarean delivery, the condition related to the reason for the admission/encounter should be selected as the principal diagnosis even if a cesarean was performed (Schraffenberger 2012, 270).

44. **d**   When subcategory codes are provided, they must be used. Code 216.1 is a subcategory code that is most specific to the diagnosis provided (Schraffenberger 2012, 3).

45. **c**   The length of multiple laceration repairs located in the same classification are added together and one code is assigned (Smith 2012, 65–66).

46. **b**   As a result of the disparity in documentation practices by providers, querying has become a common communication and educational method to advocate proper documentation practices. Queries may be made in situations where there are clinical indicators of a diagnosis but no documentation of the condition (Schraffenberger and Kuehn 2011, 345).

47. **d**   Although physicians may be contacted by phone to clarify documentation, both documentation and coding are most accurate when physicians review the health records face-to-face with coders. At the time of the review and discussion, the physician should be asked to add or modify documentation in the record. Codes should be modified, changed, or deleted only after—or when—the physician documents in the medical record (Schraffenberger and Kuehn 2011, 21).

48. **a**   In the outpatient setting, do not code a diagnosis documented as "probable." Rather, code the conditions to the highest degree of certainty for the encounter (Schraffenberger 2012, Appendix I, 81).

★ 49. **b**   Complications and comorbidities (CCs) and major complications and comorbidities (MCCs) also play a part in determining the MS-DRG. CCs and MCCs are additional, or secondary, diagnoses that ordinarily extend the length of stay. A complication is a secondary condition that arises during hospitalization; a comorbidity is one that exists at the time of admission. CCs affect many but not all MS-DRG categories. MS-DRGs are often found in sets of two or three depending on whether CCs or MCCs affect the DRG assignment. In such groupings a case with a CC would represent a higher severity level and thus would result in a higher payment than a case without a CC. A case with an MCC would be an even higher level of severity and would pay more than a case with a CC (Schraffenberger and Kuehn 2011, 201).

50. **a**   Abstracting is the process of extracting elements of data from a source document and entering them into an automated system. The purpose of this endeavor is to make those data elements available for later use. After a data element is captured in electronic form, it can be aggregated into a group of data elements to provide information needed by the user (Schraffenberger and Kuehn 2011, 425).

51. **d**   Hybrid records can affect productivity and workflow. Unless the coder is accustomed to coding from an electronic and paper record, there may be a learning curve where productivity is actually lower at first (Schraffenberger and Kuehn 2011, 287).

52. **c**   A well-trained coding staff helps ensure complete and accurate coding, which is essential for the integrity of the data collected. All coders in the facility should receive continuing education. Precise coding helps ensure compliance with regulatory requirements and helps facilitate consistency of coding in the healthcare facility. In addition, coding staff consider continuing education and training as an enhancement to their jobs. Organizations that provide continuing education take an additional step in retaining qualified coding staff (Schraffenberger and Kuehn 2011, 296).

53. **o**   Healthcare entities may design their query programs to be concurrent, retrospective, post bill, or a combination of any of these. Concurrent queries are initiated while the patient is still present. Retrospective queries are initiated after discharge and before the bill is submitted; post-bill queries are initiated after the bill has been submitted (Schraffenberger and Kuehn 2011, 347–348).

★54. **d**   Coding professionals shall adhere to the ICD coding conventions, official coding guidelines approved by the Cooperating Parties, the CPT rules established by the American Medical Association, and any other official coding rules and guidelines established for use with mandated standard code sets (Schraffenberger and Kuehn 2011, 339).

55. **a**   Present on admission is defined as present at the time the order for inpatient admission occurs—conditions that develop during an outpatient encounter, including emergency department, observation, or outpatient surgery, are considered present on admission. This patient was not admitted with a catheter-associated urinary infection and so that condition cannot be coded as POA. The patient was admitted with symptoms of a stroke and diagnoses of COPD and hypertension. The CVA was documented after admission, but the symptoms of the stroke were POA, so this condition would be coded as POA (Schraffenberger 2011, 631–632).

56. **c**   To begin the review, the coding supervisor checks the inpatient health record to ensure that the diagnosis billed as principal meets the official Uniform Hospital Discharge Data Set (UHDDS) definition for principal diagnosis. The principal diagnosis must have been a principal reason for admission, and the patient received treatment or evaluation during the stay. When several diagnoses meet all of those requirements, any of them could be selected as the principal diagnosis (Schraffenberger and Kuehn 2011, 315, 319).

57. **c** Biannual changes to ICD-9-CM codes become effective for discharges after October 1 and April 1, respectively, coinciding with the beginning and middles of the US government's fiscal year. For a patient discharged on October 5, 2011, the October 1, 2011, version of ICD-9-C would be used to code the record correctly (Schraffenberger and Kuehn 2011, 9).

58. **b** The quantitative analysis or record content review process can be handled in a number of ways. Some acute-care facilities conduct record review on a continuing basis during a patient's hospital stay. Using this method, personnel from the HIM department go to the nursing unit daily (or periodically) to review each patient's record. This type of process is usually referred to as a concurrent review because review occurs concurrently with the patient's stay in the hospital (Johns 2011, 410).

59. **d** Local coverage determination (LCD) refers to coverage rules, at a fiscal intermediary (FI) or carrier level, that provide information on what diagnoses justify the medical necessity of a test (Schraffenberger and Kuehn 2011, 461).

60. **a** Medical necessity is based on the effects of a service for the patient's physical needs and quality of life (Odom-Wesley et al. 2009, 45).

61. **c** A coding manager or physician champion should present documentation issues to educate the medical staff. General areas of concern regarding documentation should be included (Schraffenberger and Kuehn 2011, 386–387).

62. **c** Utilization management (UM) is a formal review of patient resource use. Data collected during this formal review help determine the appropriateness of the services provided. UM ensures the medical necessity of treatment provided and the cost-effective use of resources and identifies overuse or underuse of available services. Preadmission review, discharge planning, and retrospective review are all basic functions of the utilization management process. Claims management, review of potentially compensable events, and loss prevention are not basic functions of the utilization management process (Johns 2011, 650–651).

63. **a** The corporate compliance program addresses the coding function. Because the accuracy and completeness of ICD-9-CM and CPT code assignment determine the provider payment, the coding compliance program should regularly audit these codes. It is important that healthcare organizations have a strong coding compliance program (Johns 2011, 361).

64. **d** Departmental users generally have access to data only from their own department's system. If users need integrated information detailing not only their department's input, but also other parts of the record, they must request such reports through the HIM department. In its role as guardian of patient information, the HIM department tracks requests for information and ensures that a legitimate need for access to it is present (Schraffenberger and Kuehn 2011, 444–445).

65. **b** One of the elements of the auditing process is identification of risk areas. Selecting the types of cases to review is also important. Examples of various case selection possibilities include charge master description (Johns 2011, 363).

66. **c** Coding compliance activities would not include a financial incentive for coders to commit fraud. Providing a financial incentive to coders for coding claims improperly would be against any coding compliance plan and would also be a violation of AHIMA's Standards of Ethical Coding (Johns 2011, 361–364).

67. **c**   Ethical coding practices must be followed with appropriate employee counseling and remediation (Johns 2011, 26, 364).

68. **d**   Medicare does have a provision that a patient may be billed for a test that is not medically necessary if he or she receives an ABN before the test is performed. Therefore, not only must the registration staff determine whether the sign/symptom is sufficient, they may contact the patient's physician to obtain a new order or, if a new order is not provided, to issue an ABN. Success in the patient registration process involves a thoroughly educated staff with the tools to determine medical necessity, the processes in place to clarify orders, and the ability to obtain signatures on ABNs (Schraffenberger and Kuehn 2011, 467).

69. **c**   Front-end utilization management (UM) is essential to the prevention of denials for inappropriate levels of care. UM staff work with the physician to ensure that the requested services meet medical necessity requirements and are provided in the most appropriate setting. When the insurer denies the claim, an appeal may be possible. However, as mentioned above, denial management (application of the appeals process) after the fact is time-consuming and costly and does not always result in payment of the claim. UM staff are key in obtaining documentation during an inpatient stay (Schraffenberger and Kuehn 2011, 467).

70. **a**   The government and other third-party payers are concerned about potential fraud and abuse in claims processing. Therefore, ensuring that bills and claims are accurate and correctly presented is an important focus of healthcare compliance (Johns 2011, 284).

71. **d**   Policies and procedures also can be considered organizational tools. Policies are written descriptions of the organization's formal positions. Procedures are the approved methods for implementing those positions. Together, they spell out what the organization expects employees to do and how they are expected to do it (Johns 2011, 1026).

72. **b**   When an incomplete record is not rectified within a specific number of days as indicated in the medical staff rules and regulations, the record is considered to be a delinquent record. Generally, an incomplete record is considered delinquent after it has been available to the physician for completion for 15 to 30 days. The HIM department monitors the delinquent record rate very closely to ensure compliance with accrediting standards (Johns 2011, 412).

73. **b**   HIPAA allows a covered entity to adopt security protection measures that are appropriate for its organization. For example, security mechanisms will be different in complex organizations than in small organizations. Security protections in a large medical facility will be more complex than those implemented in a small group practice (Johns 2011, 1000).

74. **a**   Healthcare fraud is a deception or misrepresentation by a provider, or by representative of a provider, that may result in a false or fictitious claim for inappropriate payment by Medicare or other insurers for items or services either not rendered or rendered to a lesser extent than that described in the health record (Schraffenberger and Kuehn 2011, 370).

75. **d**   Every participating healthcare organization is subject to a periodic accreditation survey. Surveyors visit each facility and compare its programs, policies, and procedures to a prepublished set of performance standards. A key component of every accreditation survey is a review of the facility's health records. Surveyors review the documentation of patient care services to determine whether the standards for care are being met (Johns 2011, 40).

76. **c** Administered by the federal government Centers for Medicare and Medicaid Services (CMS), the Medicare Conditions of Participation or Conditions for Coverage apply to a variety of healthcare organizations that participate in the Medicare program. In other words, participating organizations receive federal funds from the Medicare program for services provided to patients and thus must follow the Medicare Conditions of Participation (Johns 2011, 109).

77. **d** Medicare-certified home healthcare also uses a standardized patient assessment instrument called the Outcomes and Assessment Information Set (OASIS). OASIS items are a component of the comprehensive assessment that is the foundation for the plan of care (Johns 2011, 100).

78. **c** Compliance with state licensing laws is required in order for healthcare organizations to begin or remain in operation within their states. To continue licensure, organizations must demonstrate their knowledge of, and compliance with, documentation regulations (Johns 2011, 108).

79. **c** The HIM department's daily ROI activities can help ensure and monitor access to patient-specific information after discharge. HIM personnel are knowledgeable in the laws and regulations governing the release of patient information. Thus, the department's ROI function is instrumental in monitoring compliance with Joint Commission standards regarding access to protected health information (Johns 2011, 460).

80. **a** Auditing information system activity is an important part of a data security program. Auditing provides a means of identifying potential access and other abuses. Auditing of an information system is performed by examining and evaluating audit trails. An audit trail is a record of system, and application activity by users. It can track when an employee has accessed the system and how long the employee has been logged into a system (Johns 2011, 926).

81. **a** Healthcare organizations are required by law to query for information on applicants requesting clinical privileges. The NPDB maintains reports on medical malpractice settlements, clinical privilege actions, and professional society membership actions against licensed healthcare providers (Shaw and Elliott 2012, 295).

82. **b** Data recovery is the process of recouping lost data or reconciling conflicting data after the system fails. These data may be from events that occurred while the system was down or from backed-up data (Sayles and Trawick 2010, 313).

83. **c** An expert system (ES) is a knowledge system built from a set of rules applied to specific problems. It can take the place of a human expert when it comes to problem solving. The system simulates the reasoning process of human experts in certain well-defined areas (Johns 2011, 881).

84. **a** Current cost: $50 × 40 calls per day = $2,000 per day × 365 days = $730,000. Cost with reduced number of help desk calls: $50 × (40 × 0.80) calls per day = $1,600 per day × 365 days = $584,000, or a savings of $146,000. Training costs of $100,000 will be recouped and a savings of $46,000 realized (Johns 2011, 1058).

85. **a** Templates ensure that the appropriate data are collected and guide users in adhering to professional practice standards. These might include nursing admission assessments, nursing progress notes, vital signs charting, intake/output records, and the like (Johns 2011, 145).

86. **c** One of the main functions of a database management system is providing security mechanisms to prevent unauthorized access and modification (Sayles and Trawick 2010, 92).

87. **d**   Clinical decision support systems (CDSS) assist healthcare providers in the actual diagnosis and treatment of patients. CDS systems integrate data from a number of systems to assist with charting, CPOE, and identifying drug contraindications. Reminders notify the healthcare provider of tests or other bits of information necessary for the healthcare provider to provide quality care. These alerts or reminders can perform a wide range of functions from indicating potential drug interactions to recommending a plan of care based on the patient's health history and clinical assessment. CDSS does not automatically transcribe medical reports (Johns 2011, 951).

88. **a**   Although sometimes used interchangeably, the terms *data* and *information* do not mean the same thing. Data represent the basic facts about people, processes, measurements, conditions, and so on. They can be collected in the form of dates, numerical measurements and statistics, textual descriptions, checklists, images, and symbols. After data have been collected and analyzed, they are converted into a form that can be used for a specific purpose. This useful form is called information. In other words, data represent facts and information represents meaning (Johns 2011, 28).

89. **a**   Discrete data entry through drop-down menus makes data entry and processing easier (Johns 2011, 145, 166).

90. **c**   An interface is a special program where specific data are identified as needing to be exchanged and then rules about how those data are structured are applied (Johns 2011, 159–160).

91. **a**   Hospitals may have applications from many different vendors, often called best of breed, meaning that a system was selected for each application that was considered to be the best in its class (Johns 2011, 176).

92. **a**   ARRA requires use of a certified EHR. This has raised considerable discussion and controversy. Since 2006, the Certification Commission for Health Information Technology (CCHIT) has been the only officially recognized certifying body for EHRs. Under HITECH, the federal government has taken on new roles with respect to certification, defining the criteria and planning for enhanced product testing to be a part of certification (Johns 2011, 153).

93. **b**   In many institutions, the chart-tracking and requisition systems are built into their automated information system. In this case, paper requisition slips are replaced by automated requisitions sent directly to the HIM department and all pertinent data are retained in a database. Automated systems such as these are similar to a library book checkout system. With an automated system, it is easy to track how many records are charged out of the HIM department at any given time, their location, and whether they have been returned on the due dates indicated (Johns 2011, 403).

94. **c**   Wide area networks (WANs) where data are transmitted across wide geographic areas generally depend on high-density trunk lines (for example, T-1 or T-3) supplied by the telephone company to transmit data. Depending on the type of phone service, the number and type of lines leased from the telephone company, and the size of the data to be transmitted, speeds and level of security can vary. Mobile telecommunications cellular network technologies, such as 3G, now provide wireless wide area network (WWAN) capability (Johns 2011, 168, 914).

95. **a**   Establishing access controls is a fundamental security strategy. Basically, the term *access control* means being able to identify which employees should have access to what data. The general practice is that employees should have access only to data they need to do their jobs. For example, an admitting clerk and a healthcare provider would not have access to the same kinds of data (Johns 2011, 992).

96. **d** Information systems must be created in a logical manner. The system development life cycle (SDLC) is the traditional way to plan and implement an IS in an organization. The major phases of the cycle are planning, analysis, design, implementation, and maintenance (Johns 2011, 882).

97. **b** The most critical resource in healthcare is patient data. The most important functions of any healthcare information system involve being able to create, modify, delete, and view patient data. And the most important storage mechanism used to perform these functions is a database. A database is an organized collection of data saved as a binary-type file on a computer. Users cannot read a binary-type file because it contains only ones and zeros. A database management system provides the ability to perform the functions already listed (Johns 2011, 902).

98. **c** Primary keys ensure that each row in a table is unique. A primary key must not change in value. Typically, a primary key is a number that is a one-up counter or a randomly generated number in large databases. A number is used because a number processes faster than an alphanumeric character. In large tables, this makes a difference. In the PATIENTS table, the PATIENT_ID is the primary key. It is good programming practice to create a primary key that is independent of the data in a table (Johns 2011, 903).

99. **b** One special form of a LAN is an intranet. An intranet is a specialized client/server network that uses Internet technologies. Intranets let corporations supply Internet services over their LANs. Essentially, intranets are private Internets with the security required to protect a corporation's assets (Johns 2011, 913).

100. **b** A run chart displays data points over a period of time to provide information about performance. The measured points of a process are plotted on a graph at regular time intervals to help team members see whether there are substantial changes in the numbers over time (Johns 2011, 623).

101. **d** The Health Plan Employer Data and Information Set (HEDIS) is sponsored by the National Committee for Quality Assurance (NCQA). HEDIS is a set of standard performance measures designed to provide healthcare purchasers and consumers with the information they need to compare the performance of managed healthcare plans. HEDIS is designed to collect administrative, claims, and health record review data. It collects standardized data about specific health-related conditions or issues so that the success of various treatment plans can be assessed and compared. HEDIS data form the basis of performance improvement (PI) efforts for health plans (Johns 2011, 210).

102. **d** Problems in patient care and other areas of the healthcare organization are usually symptoms of shortcomings inherent in a system or a process (Johns 2011, 613–614).

103. **c** The Leapfrog Group's intent is to initiate and advance safety improvements in healthcare by giving consumers more information to make healthcare choices (Shaw and Elliott 2012, 210).

104. **d** Performance improvement must be implemented with staff involved in the process. Performance improvement depends on everyone in the organization actively seeking to meet internal and external customers' spoken or anticipated needs (Johns 2011, 616–617).

105. **c** Comparing an organization's performance to the performance of other organizations that provide the same types of services is known as external benchmarking. The other organizations need not be in the same region of the country, but they should be comparable organizations in terms of patient mix and size (Shaw and Elliott 2012, 44).

106. **b** Quality measures are set and cases are identified using ICD-9-CM diagnosis codes. Acute MI is also a Core Measure. These data are monitored, rated, and ultimately compared to nationwide benchmarks to point to areas of potential improvement in patient care outcomes (Shaw and Elliott 2012, 151–152).

107. **d** Performance measurement in healthcare provides an indication of an organization's performance in relation to a specified process or outcome. Healthcare performance improvement philosophies most often focus on measuring performance in the areas of systems, processes, and outcomes. Outcomes should be scrutinized whether they are positive and appropriate or negative and diminishing (Shaw and Elliott 2012, 14).

108. **c** Establishing ground rules for meetings helps a team maintain a level of discipline. Ground rules include a discussion of attendance, time management, participation, communication, decision making, documentation, room arrangements, and clean up (Shaw and Elliott 2012, 32–33).

109. **b** Brainstorm problem areas within the current process. Brainstorming is a technique used to generate a large number of creative ideas from a group. It encourages PI team members to think "out of the box" and offer original ideas (Johns 2011, 627).

110. **a** Sampling is the recording of a smaller subset of observations of the characteristic or parameter, making certain, however, that a sufficient number of observations have been made to predict the overall configuration of the data. In this case, 82 records would be a sufficient number to review for coding quality. $(500 \times 0.05) + (480 \times 0.05) + (300 \times 0.05) + (360 \times 0.05) = 82$ records (Shaw and Elliott 2012, 46).

111. **c** An occurrence report is a structured data tool that risk managers use to gather information about potentially compensable events; also called an incident report. Effective occurrence reports carefully structure the collection of data, information, and facts in a relatively simple format (Shaw and Elliott 2012, 189).

112. **c** Every system has some degree of variation built into it. No system produces the exact same output every time. Some variations are caused by factors outside the system. This type of variation is known as special-cause variation. Similar examples of special-cause variation can be identified in our hospital systems (Johns 2011, 613–615).

113. **b** The medical staff consists of physicians who have received extensive training in various medical disciplines (internal medicine, pediatrics, cardiology, gynecology/obstetrics, orthopedics, surgery, and so on). The medical staff's primary objective is to provide high-quality patient care to the patients who come to the hospital. The medical staff is the aggregate of physicians who have been granted permission to provide clinical services in the hospital. This permission is called clinical privileges. An individual physician's privileges are limited to a specific scope of practice (Johns 2011, 711).

114. **d** The national patient safety goals outline for healthcare organizations the areas of organizational practice that most commonly lead to patient injury or other negative outcomes that can be prevented when staff utilize standardized procedures (Johns 2011, 644).

115. **c** Productivity standards should be based on both accuracy and volume. In this situation, $114 / 0.60 = 190$; $190 - 114 = 76$ more pages will need to be indexed to meet the productivity standard (Schraffenberger and Kuehn 2011, 76).

116. **c**   Whether selecting a permanent staff team or members of a team for a short-term project, making the right choice is fundamental to the team's success. Putting together a team involves understanding the challenges to be faced and considering all of the perspectives, experience, and knowledge that will be needed. The members of the team should be selected for what they can contribute to the team. Member selection should not be based purely on job title; rather, team members should be selected for the tasks that they actually can perform and the responsibilities they can carry out (Johns 2006, 1037).

117. **b**   Quality improvement organizations collaborate with practitioners, beneficiaries, providers, plans and other purchasers of healthcare services to achieve better patient care and identify areas for improvement (Johns 2011, 646).

118. **a**   An advance directive is a written document that names the patient's choice of legal representative for healthcare purposes. The person designated by the patient is then empowered to make healthcare decisions on behalf of the patient in the event that the patient is no longer capable of expressing his or her preferences. Living wills and durable powers of attorney for healthcare are two examples of advance directives (Johns 2011, 89).

119. **c**   The HIPAA Privacy Rule requires the covered entity to take certain actions when a business associate relationship is terminated. Upon notice of the termination, the covered entity needs to contact the business associate and determine if the entity still retains any protected health information from, or created for, the covered entity. The protected health information (PHI) must be destroyed, returned to the covered entity, or transferred to another business associate. Once the protected health information is transferred or destroyed, it is recommended that the covered entity obtain a certification from the business associate that either it has no protected health information , or all protected health information it had has been destroyed or returned to the covered entity (Thomason and Dennis 2008, 10).

120. **b**   The HIPAA Privacy Rule allows communications to occur for treatment purposes. The preamble repeatedly states the intent of the Rule is not to interfere with customary and necessary communications in the healthcare of the individual. Calling out a patient's name in a waiting room, or even on the facility's paging system, is considered an incidental disclosure (Thomason and Dennis 2008, 21).

121. **a**   A patient has a right to a Notice of Privacy Practices as defined in the HIPAA Privacy Rule. A healthcare provider has to provide the notice not later than the first service delivery. After that first provision of service, there is no requirement to provide a notice every time a patient receives service (Thomason and Dennis 2008, 88).

122. **c**   The HIPAA Privacy Rule defines protected health information as any individually identifiable information which is created or received by a covered entity and related to the past, present, or future physical or mental health or condition (Thomason and Dennis 2008, 89).

123. **a**   The patient can be provided a copy of his or her records, as long as he or she requests a CD and agrees to have the copies of his or her records provided on a CD or other electronic media instead of paper. However, if the patient informs that covered entity that he or she cannot read the records on a CD, the records must be provided on paper (Thomason and Dennis 2008, 91).

124. **d**   Unless a state or federal law or regulation shortens the timeframe to provide copies or access at an individual's request, the covered entity has 30 days to provide copies or access to the individual or to his or her personal representative. A covered entity may take an additional 30 days if the records are maintained off site (Thomason and Dennis 2008, 90).

125. **c**   Privacy, confidentiality, and security are related, but distinct, concepts. In the context of healthcare, privacy can be defined as the right of individuals to control access to their personal health information. Confidentiality refers to the expectation that the personal information shared by an individual with a healthcare provider during the course of care will be used only for its intended purpose. Security is the protection of the privacy of individuals and the confidentiality of health records (Johns 2011, 49).

126. **d**   Because minors are, as a general rule, legally incompetent and unable to make decisions regarding the use and disclosure of their own health information, this authority belongs to the minor's parent(s) or legal guardian(s) unless an exception applies. Generally, only one parent signature is required to authorize the use or disclosure of the minor's PHI (Brodnik 2012, 334).

127. **c**   Sometimes HITs are subpoenaed to testify as to the authenticity of the health records by confirming that they were compiled in the normal course of business and have not been altered in any way. A subpoena that is issued to elicit testimony is a subpoena *ad testificandum* (Johns 2011, 809).

128. **b**   The HIM professional should advise the medical group practice to develop a list of statutes, regulations, rules and guidelines regarding the release of the health record to be the first step in determining the components of the legal health records (Brodnik et al. 2012, 166; AHIMA e-HIM Work Group on Defining the Legal Health Record 2005).

129. **a**   Medical records, x-rays, laboratory reports, consultation reports, and other physical documents relating to the delivery of patient care are owned by the healthcare organization (Johns 2011, 803).

130. **b**   Privacy, confidentiality, and security are related, but distinct, concepts. In the context of healthcare, privacy can be defined as the right of individuals to control access to their personal health information. Confidentiality refers to the expectation that the personal information shared by an individual with a healthcare provider during the course of care will be used only for its intended purpose. Security is the protection of the privacy of individuals and the confidentiality of health records (Johns 2011, 49).

131. **d**   One of the most fundamental terms used in the Privacy Rule is *protected health information (PHI)*. The Privacy Rule defines PHI as individually identifiable health information that is transmitted by electronic media, maintained in any electronic medium, or maintained in any other form or medium (Section 164.501; Johns 2011, 821).

132. **a**   Original health records may be required by subpoena to be produced in person and the custodian of records is required to authenticate those records through testimony (Johns, 2011, 805).

133. **b**   Emancipated minors generally may authorize the access and disclosure of their own PHI. If the minor is married or previously married, the minor may authorize the disclosure or use of his or her information. If the minor is under the age of 18 and is the parent of a child, the minor may authorize the access and disclosures of his or her own information as well as that of his or her child (Brodnik 2012, 335).

134. **c**   Audit trails are usually examined by system administrators who use special analysis software to identify suspicious or abnormal system events or behavior. Because the audit trail maintains a complete log of system activity, it can also be used to help reconstruct how and when an adverse event or failure occurred (Johns 2011, 926).

135. **b**   The CDM relieves coders from coding repetitive services and supplies that require little, if any, formal documentation analysis. In these circumstances, the patient is billed automatically by linking the service to the appropriate CPT/HCPCS code (referred to as hard-coding). The advantage of hard-coding is that the code for the procedure will be reproduced accurately each time that a test, service, or procedure is ordered (Johns 2011, 354).

136. **d**   22550 has a "T" status indicator which indicates that it is a significant procedure and multiple procedure reductions will apply. In this case, there is only one CPT procedure code that is a status "T" indicator, so 100% of the fee-based APC will be paid (Casto and Layman 2011, 180).

137. **a**   A fee is a set amount or a set price. Fee-for-service means a specific payment is made for each specific service provided or rendered. The provider of the health care service charges a fee for each type of service, and the health insurance company each fee for a covered service (Casto and Layman 2011, 7–8).

138. **b**   There are two types of transfer cases under the Inpatient prospective payment system (IPPS). The first category is a patient transfer between two IPPS hospitals. A type 1 transfer is when a patient is discharged from an acute IPPS hospital (Community Hospital in this case) and is admitted to another acute IPPS hospital (Big Medical Center) on the same day. Payment is altered for the transferring hospital and is based on a per diem rate methodology. The transferring facility receives double the per diem rate for the first day plus the per diem rate for each day thereafter for the patient LOS. The receiving facility receives the full PPS payment rate for the case (Casto and Layman 2011, 129).

139. **b**   The accounts not selected for billing report is a daily report used to track the many reasons that accounts may not be ready for billing. This report is also called the discharged not final billed (DNFB) report. Accounts that have not met all facility-specified criteria for billing are held and reported on this daily tracking list. Some accounts are held because the patient has not signed the consents and authorizations required by the insurer. Still others are not billed because the primary and secondary insurance benefits have not been confirmed (Schraffenberger and Kuehn 2011, 436).

140. **c**   Indemnity plans were offered by private insurance companies that reimbursed (or indemnified) the patient for covered services up to a specified dollar limit. It was then the responsibility of the hospital to collect the money from the patient (Johns 2011, 288).

141. **b**   Private commercial insurance plans are financed through the payment of premiums. Each covered individual or family pays a preestablished amount (usually monthly), and the insurance company sets aside the premiums from all the people covered by the plan in a special fund (Johns 2011, 291).

142. **d**   Major medical insurance provides benefits up to a high-dollar limit for most types of medical expenses. However, it usually requires patients to pay large deductibles. It also may place limits on charges (for example, room and board) and require patients to pay a portion of the expenses (Johns 2011, 288).

143. **a**   Medicare Part A covers inpatient hospital care, some skilled nursing care, home health care and hospice care. Dental services are not covered under Medicare Part A (Johns 2011, 294).

144. **c**   A benefit period begins on the day of admission and ends when the beneficiary has been out of the hospital for 60 days in a row, including the day of discharge. In this case, the first benefit period began on 1/1 (Johns 2011, 295).

145. **c**   Healthcare fraud is defined as an intentional representation that an individual knows to be false or does not believe to be true and makes, knowing that the representation could result in some unauthorized benefit to himself or herself or some other person. An example of fraud is billing for a service that was not furnished. The other three options are acceptable practices for healthcare organizations to use to effectively manage their revenue cycles (Casto and Layman 2011, 34–35).

146. **a**   A benefit cap is an overarching limitation and is also known as a maximum dollar plan limit. A benefit cap is the total dollar amount that the healthcare insurance policy will pay for the policyholder and each covered dependent for covered healthcare services during a specified period, such as a year or lifetime (Casto and Layman 2011, 68).

147. **c**   Although the principal owner of the CDM is the finance department in most instances, maintaining the CDM is a joint responsibility. Ideally, updating and maintaining the CDM is the work of a team or committee that includes members from the finance, patient accounting, information systems, HIM department, and managers of clinical departments, such as laboratory or radiology (Schraffenberger and Kuehn 2011, 234).

148. **d**   A CDI program provides a mechanism for the coding staff to communicate with the physician regarding nonspecific diagnostic statements or when additional diagnoses are suspected but not clearly stated in the record which helps to avoid assumption coding (Schraffenberger and Kuehn 2011, 356).

149. **a**   Healthcare fraud is a deception or misrepresentation by a provider, or by a representative of a provider, that may result in a false or fictitious claim for inappropriate payment by Medicare or other insurers for items or services either not rendered or rendered to a lesser extent than that described in the claim. In other words, healthcare fraud is the submission of a claim for payment of items or services that the person knew—or should have known—were not provided (Schraffenberger and Kuehn 2011, 370).

150. **a**   The health information manager must continuously promote complete, accurate, and timely documentation to ensure appropriate coding, billing, and reimbursement. This requires a close working relationship with the medical staff, perhaps through the use of a physician champion. Physician champions assist in educating medical staff members on documentation needed for accurate billing. The medical staff is more likely to listen to a peer than to a facility employee, especially when the topic is documentation needed to ensure appropriate reimbursement (Schraffenberger and Kuehn 2011, 381).

121/150 = 81%

−29

121

Exam 2

1. **a** In 1997, the Centers for Disease Control and Prevention (CDC) through its National Center for Injury Prevention and Control (NCIPC) published a data set called Data Elements for Emergency Department Systems (DEEDS). The purpose of this data set is to support the uniform collection of data in hospital-based emergency departments and to reduce incompatibilities in emergency department records (Johns 2011, 211).

2. **a** To support the development of networked health information systems, NHIN defines three dimensions of the infrastructure that provide a means for conceptualizing the capture, storage, communication, processing, and presentation of information for each group of information users. Core content of the personal health dimensions include treatment plans and instructions (Johns 2011, 213–214).

3. **d** Filing accuracy can be checked by conducting a random audit of the storage area. To conduct a study, a section of the permanent file room can be checked for misfiles. Any files found or noted and a filing accuracy rate can be determined and compared against the established standard. In this scenario, there were 527 instances of accurate filing out of 540 sampled: (527 / 540) × 100 = 97.6% (Johns 2011, 417).

4. **c** Outcomes and Assessment Information Set (OASIS) is a standardized data set designed to gather data about Medicare beneficiaries who are receiving services from a home health agency. OASIS contains more than 30 new data elements including activities of daily living (ADL) (Johns 2011, 209).

5. **a** A data dictionary is a descriptive list of the data elements to be collected in an information system or database whose purpose is to ensure consistency of terminology (Johns 2011, 1125).

6. **d** Several factors must be addressed when assessing data quality. These include: data accuracy, consistency completeness and timeliness. Cost to process the data does not influence the quality (Johns 2011, 508–509).

7. **c** If during record analysis, missing or incomplete information is identified, and HIM personnel can issue deficiency notification(s) to the appropriate caregiver to assure the completeness of the health record (Odom-Wesley et al. 2009, 250).

8. **d** Data precision is the term used to describe expected data values. As part of data definition, the acceptable values or value ranges for each data element must be defined. For example, a precise data definition related to gender would include three values: male, female, and unknown (Johns 2011, 48).

9. **b** Documentation of medical history, consents, and the physical examination must be available in the patient's record before any surgical procedures may be performed (Odom-Wesley et al. 2009, 108).

10. **a** The operative report describes the surgical procedures performed on the patient. Each report typically includes the name of the surgeon and assistants, date, duration and description of the procedure, preoperative and postoperative diagnosis, estimated blood loss, descriptions of any unusual or unique events during the course of the surgery, normal and abnormal findings, as well as any specimens that were removed (Johns 2011, 73).

11. **c**   Many hospitals incorporate documents into their electronic health record systems. Digital scanners create images of handwritten and printed documents that are then store in health record databases as electronic files. Using scanned images solves many of the problems associated with traditional paper-based health records and hybrid records (Odom-Wesley et al. 2009, 227).

12. **a**   An off-site storage company is usually a contracted service that stores health records. For a fee, the company then retrieves and delivers records requested by the healthcare facility's HIM department. Because the records are filed in boxes, each box needs a unique identifier so it can be located. The records in each box must be identified and cross-indexed to the box in which they are stored (Johns 2011, 401).

13. **c**   Filing accuracy can be checked by conducting a random audit of the storage area. To conduct a study, a section of the permanent file room can be checked for misfiles. Any files found or noted and a filing accuracy rate can be determined and compared against the established standard. In this scenario, there was a 7% error rate for the 10,000 records filed in the sample. If the cost of each misfile is $200, this would cost the facility $140,000, ($10,000 $\times$ 0.07) $\times$ $200 = $140,000 (Johns 2011, 417).

14. **d**   Review of body systems is typically documented in the report of a physical examination. This would include documentation regarding the HEENT (head, eyes, ears, nose, and throat) and the chest (Johns 2011, 65).

15. **b**   Cancer registries are typically maintained by hospitals on a voluntary basis or by state law. Many states require that hospitals report their data to a central state-wide registry or incidence surveillance program who in turn reports the data to the Centers for Disease Control (CDC) (Brodnik 2012, 392–393).

16. **c**   The productivity increase with telecommuting is 20%. The facility has five coders that are currently coding 100 charts a day. With this 20% increase, the existing five coders can code four records more per day each (a 20% increase). 24 $\times$ 5 = 120. If the discharges increase by 44 charts, the facility would need one more FTE in the telecommuting staffing model, since each coder can code 24 records/day (Johns 2011, 1063–1065).

17. **a**   2 (# of records per hour) $\times$ 2,080 = 4160 records per FTE. 12,500 / 4,160 = 3.0 employees (Johns 2011, 1060–1062).

18. **a**   The MPI is a list or database created or maintained by a healthcare facility to record the name and identification number of every patient who has ever been admitted or treated in the facility (Johns 2011, 1147).

19. **d**   There are a variety of factors that influence the quality of data maintained on patients, clients and residents of healthcare organizations that is related to specific encounters in which the care was provided. These include case-mix management, length of inpatient stay, professional fee billing versus facility billing, data abstract type, and health record documentation (Schraffenberger and Kuehn 2011, 258–259).

20. **a**   The types of data elements that are abstracted, or defined as indexed fields in an automated system, vary from facility to facility. Generally, however, any data elements that are needed for selecting cases for reports must be abstracted or indexed. Some of the typical data fields that can be searched for the purpose of finding and reporting include: patient name, zip code, health records number, patient account number, attending physician, etc. (Schraffenberger and Kuehn 2011, 426–427).

21. **b** Aggregate data is data extracted from individual health records and combined to form de-identified information about groups of patients that can be compared and analyzed (Schraffenberger and Kuehn 2011, 424–425, 517).

22. **a** Department managers frequently use the CDM as a tool to accumulate workload statistics. Workload statistics can assist managers with the tasks of monitoring productivity and provide data regarding resources used, such as equipment, personnel, services and supplies (Schraffenberger and Kuehn 2011, 223).

23. **c** A line graph may be used to display time trends. A line graph is especially useful for plotting a large number of observations. It also allows several sets of data to be presented on one graph (Johns 2011, 540–543).

24. **b** The denominator (the number of times an event could have occurred) in this case would be 263 as 263 women delivered (Johns 2011, 526).

25. **d** The average daily census is the average number of inpatients treated during a given period of time; there are 30 days in September, so 3,000 / 30 = 100 (Johns 2011, 548).

26. **b** The average length of stay is the mean length of stay of hospital inpatients discharged during a given period of time. Add the total days for each patient and divide by 9 = 6 days (Johns 2011, 553).

27. **d** Demographic data is used to identify an individual, such as name, address, gender, age, and other information linked to a specific person (Johns 2011, 487, 1126).

28. **d** A hospital can monitor its performance under the MS-DRG system by monitoring its case-mix index (CMI). The CMI is the average of the relative weights of all cases treated at a given hospital. The Medicare CMI for every participating hospital is published annually in the *Federal Register*. The CMI can be used to make comparisons between hospitals and to assess the quality of documentation and coding at a particular hospital (Schraffenberger and Kuehn 2011, 204).

29. **d** Record retention should only be done in accordance with federal and state law and written retention and destruction policies of the organization. AHIMA's recommended retention standards for master patient index (MPI) is permanent retention (Johns 2011, 406).

30. **c** A variation on open-shelf files is the mobile or compact file. Instead of having aisle space between every row of files, mobile files conserve floor space by providing only one aisle of space. This is accomplished by mounting the file shelves on tracks secured to the floor. The shelves then are moved by hand, with mechanical assistance, or electronically. This type of storage system is ideal in facilities where storage space is a major concern (Johns 2011, 396–397).

31. **a** The coding function must be reviewed on a ongoing basis for consistency and accuracy. Coding processed should be monitored for elements of quality. One of these elements is reliability. Reliability is the degree to which the same results are achieved consistently (that is, when different individuals code the same health record, they assign the same codes) (Johns 2011, 265).

32. **a** Volume 1 of ICD-9-CM contains 17 chapters that classify conditions according to etiology or by specific anatomical system. These categories are 001–999.9 (Schraffenberger 2012, 2–3).

33. **c** Resolving failed edits is one of many duties of the HIM department. Various medical departments depend on the coding expertise of HIM professionals to avoid incorrect coding and potential compliance issues (Schraffenberger and Kuehn 2011, 237–238).

34. **a** Two indicators of coder's skill are accuracy and volume. Productivity standards should be based on both accuracy and volume (Schraffenberger and Kuehn 2011, 76).

35. **c** Presentations on complex MS-DRGs should include the etiology and manifestations of conditions, along with related complications. For example, a presentation on MS-DRGs 870–872, septicemia or severe sepsis, with or without mechanical ventilation over 96 hours, with or without MCC, could include the difference between sepsis, urosepsis, and a urinary tract infection. The presentation also would include the etiology and manifestations for sepsis, abnormal lab values, coding guidelines and treatment options (Schraffenberger and Kuehn 2011, 297).

36. **d** According to the American Hospital Association's Central Office on ICD-9-CM, ICD-9-CM is used for classification of morbidity and mortality for statistical purposes, reporting of diagnoses by physicians and many more users. But, ICD-9-CM is not used to identify supplies, products and services provided to patients (Johns 2011, 239).

37. **d** The HIM department can plan focused review based on specific problem areas after the initial baseline review has been completed. Some potential problem coding areas for focused reviews include: controversial issues identified in AHA *Coding Clinic*, recent data quality issues identified by external review agencies and analysis of comparison data. APC groups would not be part of a focused inpatient audit (Schraffenberger and Kuehn 2011, 314–315).

38. **d** Coding managers play an important role in the data quality review and educational process for coders. They are responsible for developing action plans for individual coders (Schraffenberger and Kuehn 2011, 313).

39. **a** ICD-9-CM is published in three volumes. Volume 1 is known as the Tabular List. It contains the numerical listing of codes that represent diseases and injuries. Volume 2 is the Alphabetic Index. It consists of an Alphabetic Index for all the codes listed in Volume 1. The Tabular List and Alphabetic Index for Procedures are published as Volume 3. There is no Volume 4 (Johns 2011, 239–240).

40. **a** Directly below a category or subcategory code: The instructions in the inclusion note apply to all codes within the range. Because the inclusion note is not repeated, the coder must look back to the beginning of the subcategory, category, section, or chapter to ensure that important instructions are not missed (Schraffenberger 2012, 17–18).

41. **a** Assign code 996.41, Mechanical loosening of prosthetic joint, for the loosening of the acetabular component. Assign code V43.64, Organ or tissue replaced by other means, hip, to identify the prosthetic joint associated with the mechanical complication. Assign code 00.71, Revision hip replacement, acetabular component, for the hip prosthesis. Code 00.75, Revision hip replacement bearing surface, metal on metal, should be assigned as an additional procedure to identify the specific type of bearing surface (Schraffenberger 2012, 35).

42. **b** 434.90 is used because the type of cerebral artery occlusion is unspecified; 342.90 is used because the side affected by the hemiparesis in not indicated in the diagnosis; 784.3 codes the aphasia; 401.9 is used because the hypertension is unspecified as to whether it is malignant or benign (Schraffenberger 2012, 35, 198).

43. **c** Colonoscopy includes examining the transverse colon. Proctosigmoidoscopy involves examining the rectum and sigmoid colon. Sigmoidoscopy involves examining the rectum, sigmoid colon and may include portion of the descending colon (Smith 2012, 117).

44. **c** The hospital-acquired conditions (HAC) provision is an additional component of pay-for-performance utilizing reported ICD-9-CM diagnosis codes and the present-on-admission (POA) indicator to identify quality issues. Pressure ulcers not present on admission or identified with the POA indicator on the claim would not be paid for as a CC or MCC because they would be considered an HAC (Casto and Layman 2011, 283).

45. **c** A complication is a secondary condition that arises during hospitalization; a comorbidity is one that exists at the time of admission (Schraffenberger and Kuehn 2011, 201).

46. **c** Each HCPCS code is assigned to one and only one APC. The APC assignment for a procedure or services does not change based on the patient's medical condition or the severity of illness. There may be an unlimited number of APCs per encounter for a single patient. The number of APC assignments is based on the number of reimbursable procedures or services provided for that patient. In this instance, the patient has five APCs (Casto and Layman 2011, 180).

47. **a** CHF is the principal diagnosis and must be sequenced first (Schraffenberger 2012, 66).

48. **d** Hematuria is an adverse effect as opposed to a poisoning because it was correctly prescribed and correctly taken (Schraffenberger 2012, 377).

49. **a** This is an example of a circumstance where the chronic condition must be verified. All secondary conditions must match the definition in the UHDDS and whether the COPD does is not clear (Schraffenberger 2012, 71).

50. **b** The placenta previa is the reason for the C-section and therefore is the principal diagnosis (Schraffenberger 2012, 270).

51. **b** The principal diagnosis determines the MDC assignment (Johns 2011, 322).

52. **d** The weight of each DRG is multiplied by the number of discharges for that DRG to arrive at the total weight for each DRG—in this situation 15,192. The total weights are summed and divided by the number of total discharges to arrive at the case-mix index for a hospital: 15,192 / 10,471 = 1.45 (Johns 2011, 324).

53. **c** MS-DRG 193 has the highest weight and therefore would have the highest payment (Johns 2011, 323).

54. **a** The Outpatient Code Editor (OCE) is a software program linked to the Correct Coding Initiative that applies a set of logical rules to determine whether various combinations of codes are correct and appropriately represent the services provided (Johns 2011, 348).

55. **b** A complication is a secondary condition that arises during hospitalization; a comorbidity is one that exists at the time of admission (Schraffenberger and Kuehn 2011, 201).

56. **c**   Managing remote staff presents new considerations. It is not necessarily more difficult to manage remote staff; rather, it presents different challenges. In the remote environment, managers may need to rely on productivity and coding accuracy reports to determine the success of remote employees. When allowing coders to work from home or contracting with remote coders, work expectations must be established in advance (Schraffenberger and Kuehn 2011, 92–93).

57. **c**   Reporting options for POA assignment are: Y—present at the time of inpatient admission, N—not present at the time of inpatient admission, U—documentation is insufficient to determine if condition was present on admission, W—provider is unable to clinically determine whether condition was present on admission (Schraffenberger 2012, Appendix I, 83–84).

58. **b**   One of the elements of the auditing process is identification of risk areas. Some major risk areas include Chargemaster description, medical necessity, MS-DRG coding accuracy, variations in case mix, etc. Admission diagnosis and complaints, clinical laboratory results and radiology orders are not risk areas that should be targeting for audit (Johns 2011, 363).

59. **d**   The ability to copy previous entries and paste into a current entry lead to a record in which a clinician may, upon signing the documentation, unwittingly swear to the accuracy and comprehensiveness of substantial amounts of duplicated or inapplicable information as well as the incorporation of misleading or erroneous documentation. The HIM professional plays a critical role in developing policies and procedures to ensure the integrity of patient information (Odom-Wesley et al. 2009, 266; Johns 2011, 777).

60. **c**   There are two areas which are consistently identified by the OIG as being responsible for 70% of bad claims; one is insufficient or missing documentation, and the other is failure to document medical necessity appropriately which would include the claims submission process (Brodnik et al. 2012, 443–444).

61. **d**   The use of colored paper or ink other than black, or shading of text in EDMS should be minimized or eliminated because the color can adversely affect the quality of scanned images (Johns 2011, 415).

62. **b**   Unacceptable documentation practices include back-dating progress notes or other documentation in the patient's record and changing the documentation to reflect the known outcomes of care. The professional Code of Ethics requires the HIM professional to assure accurate and timely documentation (Johns 2011, 778)

63. **a**   Utilization controls include the prospective and retrospective review of the healthcare services planned for, or provided to, patients. For example, a prospective utilization review of a plan to hospitalize a patient for minor surgery might determine the surgery could be safely performed less expensively in an outpatient setting. Prospective utilization review often called precertification and is done in managed fee-for-service reimbursement (Johns 2011, 316).

64. **b**   Ongoing evaluation is critical to successful coding and billing for third-party payer reimbursement. In the past, the goal of internal audit programs was to increase revenues for the provider. Today, the goal is to protect providers from sanctions or fines. Healthcare organizations can implement monitoring programs by conducting regular, periodic audits of (1) ICD-9-CM and CPT/HCPCS coding and (2) claims development and submission. In addition, audits should be conducted to follow up on previous reviews that resulted in the identification of problems (for example, poor coding quality or errors in claims submission) (Johns 2011, 362).

65. c According to the Health Care Quality Improvement Act of 1986, facilities are required to report professional review actions such as malpractice, disciplinary actions, and credentialing information on physicians, dentists, and other facility-based practitioners to the National Practitioner Data Bank (Brodnik et al. 2012, 387–388).

66. c The primary role of the case manager is to coordinate and facilitate care. The care-planning process extends beyond the acute-care setting to ensure the patient receives appropriate follow-up services. Many healthcare insurers and managed care organizations also employ case managers to coordinate medical care and ensure the medical necessity of the services provided to beneficiaries (Johns 2011, 651).

67. c Coding usually determines a facility's reimbursement for services rendered, it is a high-risk area that should be continuously monitored to ensure compliance with all applicable regulations. Coding compliance plans are implemented to demonstrate the steps being taken to ensure correct coding (Schraffenberger and Kuehn 2011, 382–383).

68. c Operation Restore Trust was released in 1995 to target fraud and abuse among healthcare providers. The major push for accurate coding and billing eventually spread to be a nationwide effort (Casto and Layman 2011, 36).

69. d Over the past several years, the OIG has published several site-of-service documents to help providers develop internal compliance programs that include elements for ensuring compliance. One of the elements included is written policies and procedures (Schraffenberger and Kuehn 2011, 376–377).

70. c Abuse occurs when a healthcare provider unknowingly or unintentionally submits an inaccurate claim for payment. Abuse generally results from unsound medical, business, or fiscal practices that directly or indirectly result in unnecessary costs to the Medicare program. An example of abuse involves inadvertently reporting a procedure code that describes a service that was more extensive than the procedure performed (Casto and Layman 2011, 34–35).

71. c All patient medical record entries must be legible, complete, dated, timed, and authenticated in written or electronic form by the person responsible for providing or evaluating the service provided, consistent with hospital policies and procedures (Electronic Code of Federal Regulations 2012).

72. c Over the past several years, OIG has published several site-of-service documents to help providers develop internal compliance programs that include the seven elements for ensuring compliance as outlined in the US Sentencing Guidelines in 1991 (Schraffenberger and Kuehn 2011, 376–377).

73. d In an effort to provide structure and accountability to this important process, HIM departments have implemented coding compliance plans to demonstrate the steps being taken to ensure data quality. The coding compliance plan should be based on the same principles as those of the corporate program (Schraffenberger and Kuehn 2011, 382–383).

74. b Customized letters are critical to the ROI system. Customized letters and forms may be used to communicate with the requestor for many purposes including a letter notifying the individual making a request that the authorization is invalid (Sayles and Trawick 2010, 185–186).

75. **c**   The chart location system is designed to track the paper medical record. This tracking is important because paper records are moved from place to place for patient care, quality reviews, coding, and many other purposes. The Joint Commission regulations require medical records to be readily accessible for patient care. The chart locator supports that mandate (Sayles and Trawick 2010, 193–195).

76. **a**   Accreditation standards are developed to reflect reasonable quality standards. The performance of each participating organization is evaluated annually against the standards. The accreditation process is voluntary; healthcare organizations choose to participate in order to improve the care they provide to their patients (Johns 2011, 679).

77. **c**   A knowledge management system (KMS) is a more recent type of information system that has the potential to increase work effectiveness. This type of system supports the creation, organization, and dissemination of business or clinical knowledge and expertise to providers, employees, and managers throughout the healthcare enterprise (Johns 2011, 881).

78. **a**   Health record retention policies depend on a number of factors. They must comply with local, state, and federal statutes and regulations. Retention regulations vary by state and possibly by organization type. Health records should be retained for at least the period specified by the state's statute of limitations for malpractice, and other claims must be taken into consideration when determining the length of time to retain records as evidence (Johns 2011, 815).

79. **b**   HIPAA requires the devices and media on which data are stored be protected. This requires policies and procedures that ensure that disks, tapes, and videos are physically protected from harm or intrusion. Essentially, the organization must have controls for tracking the access, removal, and disposal of hardware and software (Johns 2011, 1004–1005).

80. **c**   The first and most fundamental strategy is to establish a security organization that is responsible for managing all aspects of computer security. This usually involves appointing someone in the organization to coordinate the development of security policies and to ensure that they are followed (Johns 2011, 988).

81. **a**   Audit controls are required by HIPAA. One method of monitoring is the use of audit trails. Audit trails are a recording of activities occurring in an information system. Audit trails can monitor system level controls such as who logs on, when the log on, and applications accessed. Application level controls track what systems they used, what the user saw, and what they did (Sayles and Trawick 2010, 323–324).

82. **d**   Demographics is the study of the statistical characteristics of human populations. In the context of healthcare, demographic information includes the following elements: patient's full name, patient's facility identification or account number, patient's address, patient's telephone number, patient's date and place of birth, patient's gender, patient's race or ethnic origin, patient's marital status, name and address of patient's next of kin, date and time of admission, hospital's name, address, and telephone number (Johns 2011, 84–85).

83. **a**   Clinical decision support systems (CDSS) assist healthcare providers in the actual diagnosis and treatment of patients. CDS systems integrate data from a number of systems to assist with charting, CPOE, and identifying drug contraindications (Johns 2011, 951).

84. **d**   In healthcare organizations, computer-based information systems are used to help managers at different levels to do their work. The managers of the nursing, physical therapy, and health information management (HIM) departments often use computer systems called management information systems (MISs) to manage budgets, create work schedules, perform employee evaluations, and so on (Johns 2011, 877).

85. **b**   To ensure essential information is not omitted, essential data field should be required. A template can be used as an effective way to ensure the appropriate data are collected and guide users in adhering to professional practice standards. These might include nursing admission assessments, nursing progress notes, vital signs charting, intake/output records, and the like (Johns 2011, 145).

86. **c**   An information system (IS) is the integration of several elements of a business process to achieve a specific outcome. The system receives and processes input and provides output (Johns 2011, 875).

87. **a**   A transaction-processing system (TPS) is an example of an operations support system. A TPS manages the different kinds of transactions that occur in a healthcare facility. Patient admissions, employee time cards, and supply purchases are examples of transactions that take place in a healthcare facility (Johns 2011, 878).

88. **b**   Organizations use multiple databases in their daily business operations. Many of these are separated from each other and the data are not available in a consolidated form to help managers and others make decisions. A data warehouse is a special type of database that alleviates this problem by consolidating and storing data from various databases throughout the enterprise (Johns 2011, 909).

89. **c**   Most hospitals and other healthcare facilities use computer systems for registering patients and tracking their encounters that require multiple points for data input. Within hospitals, these systems are commonly known as admission-discharge-transfer (ADT) systems or registration-admission-discharge-transfer (R-ADT) systems. Diagnostic and length of stay (LOS) information also can be stored in ADT systems (Johns 2011, 947).

90. **c**   A primary key must uniquely identify a record. None of the options provided will uniquely identify a record. Multiple individuals may have the same name and birth dates (Johns 2011, 903).

91. **b**   Templates ensure that the appropriate data are collected and guide users in adhering to professional practice standards. These might include nursing admission assessments, nursing progress notes, vital signs charting, intake/output records, and the like. Templates include drop-down menus, checkboxes, type-ahead, and other data entry aids. They are not static, however. A considerable amount of logic is built into an automated template so they adjust to the patient's gender, reason for visit, or chief complaint, and reflect guidelines established for the proper documentation established for different conditions (Johns 2011, 145).

92. **a**   Prototyping is another analysis technique. A prototype is a model or example of what a completed IS may look like. Prototyping a system allows for maximum end-user input while speeding up the analysis and development process. End users and analysts work together to develop the external features of the IS, such as input screens and reports. These external features provide the look and feel of the proposed system but do not include actual program application codes that would make the IS work (Johns 2011, 885).

93. **a**   Thorough testing of new systems (hardware and/or software) before the actual conversion date is critical. Systems testers test the use cases developed in the design phase against the system's requirements. If a requirement fails, the tester reports the problem to the technical staff. The technical staff then fixes the problem and completes their report. Based on this report, the testers retest the requirement until it passes. Testing should be conducted using actual patient data, not sample data the vendor has provided or the organization has created for training purposes. Correcting a problem in the test mode is often easier than correcting it after the system is fully operational (Johns 2011, 890).

94. **a**   Most organizations create an EHR steering committee to engage all the various stakeholders in EHR planning and development. This ensures that the EHR planning is comprehensive and also starts the process of introducing change and gaining buy-in (Johns 2011, 175).

95. **b**   Data security embodies three basic concepts: protecting the privacy of data, ensuring the integrity of data, ensuring the availability of data (Johns 2011, 984).

96. **c**   Edit checks help to ensure data integrity by allowing only reasonable and predetermined values to be entered into the computer (Johns 2011, 992).

97. **b**   In the HIPAA Security Rule, one of the technical safeguards standards is access control. This includes automatic log-off, which ensures electronics processes that terminate an electronic session after a predetermined time of inactivity (Brodnik et al. 2012, 307).

98. **a**   Data models provide a contextual framework and graphical representation that aid in the definition of data elements. In a relational database, the data model lays the foundation for the database and identifies important entities, their attributes and the relationships among entities (Johns 2002) An entity is anything about which data can be stored and can be a concept, person, place, thing, or event. In the cancer registry example above, "PATIENT" and "CASES" would both be entities (Johns 2011, 139, 904).

99. **a**   Clinical decision support (CDS) systems assist healthcare providers in the actual diagnosis and treatment of patients. CDS systems integrate data from a number of systems to assist with charting, CPOE, and identifying drug contraindications. Reminders notify the healthcare provider of tests or other information necessary for the healthcare provider to provide quality care. These alerts or reminders can perform a wide range of functions from indicating potential drug interactions to recommending a plan of care based on the patient's health history and clinical assessment (Johns 2011, 951).

100. **b**   The Joint Commission introduced the ORYX initiative to integrate outcomes data and other performance measurement data into its accreditation processes. The goal of the ORYX initiative is to integrate outcomes and other performance measures into the accreditation process through data collection about specific core measures (Johns 2011, 211–212).

101. **c**   Performance improvement is based on several fundamental principles, including: the structure of a system determines its performance, all systems demonstrate variation, improvements rely on the collection and analysis of data that increase knowledge, PI requires the commitment and support of top administration, PI works best when leaders and employees know and share the organization's mission, vision, and values, PI efforts take time to require a big investment in people, excellent teamwork is essential, communication must be open, honest and multidirectional, success must be celebrated to encourage more success. Identifying and reprimanding individuals responsible for quality problems is not a principle of contemporary performance improvement (Johns 2011, 613–614).

102. **a** To be successful in implementing PI programs, healthcare organizations may have to restructure and create a new culture to accommodate the enormous changes and competition that exist in today's healthcare environment. Changes in customer expectations and the way that healthcare is financed may demand organizational restructuring. PI must be encompassed in an environment of cooperation. It is most successful in organizations that have an interdisciplinary and participative management approach. As discussed previously, shared vision is one of the cornerstones of a successful PI program. A shared vision puts everyone, including the governing board, upper management, and employees on the same path to organizational success. Changing to a shared leadership environment can create a new organizational culture of shared vision, responsibility, and accountability (Johns 2011, 638).

103. **b** There are many groups trying to improve patient safety. There are a number of organizations (governmental, private, and not-for-profit) that are engaged in patient safety issues. Some of these organizations are: Institute for Healthcare Improvement, Commonwealth Fund, Leapfrog Group, and many others. Safe Practices for All is not an example of one (Brodnik et al. 2012, 474)

104. **b** The contemporary approach to PI is much more proactive than the traditional quality management approach. Although PI uses several traditional quality management techniques such as quality indicators, most often its primary focus is on continually making small, targeted changes for improvement, which over time lead to significant overall improvement. Performance improvement is not a philosophy that is satisfied with the status quo; it is not based on the "if it isn't broke, don't fix it" assumption. Nor does PI operate on the theory of identifying "bad apples," where one conducts inspections to identify defects (Johns 2011, 610).

105. **d** Characteristics for data entry should be uniform throughout the patient record to ensure consistency. Abbreviations are extremely easy to use; however, data must have definitions and be uniform. Otherwise, problems can arise from this inconsistency (Sayles and Trawick 2010, 83–84).

106. **c** In addition to documenting meeting activities, the PI team must provide regular reports to the organization's PI and Patient Safety Council. Quarterly reports should be submitted to the organization's PI and Patient Safety Council (Shaw and Elliott, 2012, 71).

107. **a** When an organization compares its current performance to its own internal historical data, or uses data from similar external organizations, it helps establish an organization benchmark. A benchmark is a systematic comparison of one organization's measure characteristics of those of another similar organization (Johns 2011, 618).

108. **a** When a team examines a process with the intention of making improvements, it must first understand the process thoroughly. Each team member has a unique perspective and significant insight about how a portion of the process works. Flow charts help all the team members understand the process in the same way (Johns 2011, 626–627).

109. **b** The credentialing and privileging process for the initial appointment and reappointment of independent practitioners should be defined in the healthcare organizations medical staff bylaws and should be uniformly applied (Shaw and Elliott 2012, 294).

110. **b** One of the common quality improvement tools used for risk management purposes is the cause and effect diagram. A cause-and-effect diagram facilitates root–cause analysis. The diagram is sometimes called a fishbone diagram because of its characteristic shape (Johns 2011, 628–629).

111. **a**   Performance improvement is based on several fundamental principles, including: the structure of a system determines its performance; all systems demonstrate variation; improvements rely on the collection and analysis of data that increase knowledge; PI requires the commitment and support of top administration; PI works best when leaders and employees know and share the organization's mission, vision, and values; PI efforts take time to require a big investment in people; excellent teamwork is essential; communication must be open, honest, and multidirectional; success must be celebrated to encourage more success. Teamwork is not an optional element of performance improvement. It is an essential element (Johns 2011, 613–614).

112. **c**   Once a benchmark for each performance measure is determined, analyzing data collection results becomes more meaningful. Often, further study or more focused data collection on a performance measure is triggered when data collection results fall outside the established benchmark. When variation is discovered or when unexpected events suggest performance problems, members of the organization may decide there is an opportunity for improvement (Shaw and Elliott 2012, 7).

113. **b**   Reviewing for deficiencies is an example of quantitative analysis. The goal of quantitative analysis to is make sure there are no missing reports, forms, or required signatures in a patient record. Timely completion of this process ensures a complete health record (Johns 2011, 409–410).

114. **b**   Process indicators measure the actions by which services are provided, the things people or devices do, from conducting appropriate tests, to making a diagnosis, to actually carrying out a treatment (Johns 2011, 610).

115. **c**   The team must answer this question: Why has this team been formed? The team must define its mission in order to create a "map" or plan of the means by which it will examine the issues and plan its activities (Johns 2011, 626).

116. **a**   Collecting data on current performance and tasks allows the HIM supervisor to include all tasks that are being performed in the new job descriptions. When more than one person is performing a task, the data could be collected over time and averaged. The experience and overall performance of each person must be considered in setting the standard (Johns 2011, 1064).

117. **d**   Most performance improvement methodologies recognize that the organization must identify and continuously monitor the important organizational and patient-focused functions that they perform, with special emphasis on high-volume, high-risk, and problem-prone outcomes (Shaw and Elliott 2012, 15).

118. **b**   One of the major purposes of a health record is that it is the legal business record of an organization and serves as evidence in lawsuits or other legal actions. It is the record that is used for legal purposes and would be the record released upon a valid request (Brodnik et al. 2012, 165).

119. **a**   The basic principles of health record documentation apply to both paper-based and electronic patient records. Changes to health records are acceptable, if done according to documentation guidelines (Johns 2011, 1007).

120. **b**   Associated with ownership of health records is the legal concept of the custodian of records. The custodian of health records is the individual who has been designated as having responsibility for the care, custody, control, and proper safekeeping and disclosure of health records (Brodnik et al. 2012, 7–8).

121. **b** The individual who brings a lawsuit is the plaintiff. The individual or company that is the object of the lawsuit is the defendant. The plaintiff begins the lawsuit by filing a complaint in court (Johns 2011, 809).

122. **b** If the paper medical record is destroyed, the imaging record would be the legal health record. This may not be the case if the paper record is retained. State laws typically view the original medical record as the legal record when it is available. Those who choose to destroy the original medical record may do so within weeks, months, or years of scanning. If the record was destroyed according to guidelines for destruction and no scanned record exists, the certificate of destruction should be presented in lieu of the record (Sayles and Trawick 2010, 154).

123. **b** The responsibilities of the health information management (HIM) professional include a wide range of functions and activities. Regardless of the employer—such as healthcare facility, vendor, pharmaceutical company, or research firm—the HIM professional's core ethical obligations are to protect patient privacy and confidential information and communication and to assure security of that information (Johns 2011, 752).

124. **d** A firewall is a part of a computer system or network that is designed to block unauthorized access while permitting authorized communications. It is a software program or device that filters information between two networks, usually between a private network like an intranet and a public network like the Internet (Johns 2011, 922).

125. **c** Maintaining all interim reports provides the greatest measure of security. Managing health information in a hybrid record environment is challenging, but by maintaining the reports the facility will reduce some potential problems (AHIMA E-HIM Taskforce Report 2010, "Managing the Transition from Paper to EHRs," updated November 2010).

126. **b** Beneficence would require the HIM professional to ensure that the information is released only to individuals who need it to do something that will benefit the patient (for example, to an insurance company for payment of a claim) (Johns 2011, 752).

127. **d** A subpoena *duces tecum* instructs the recipient to bring documents and other records with himself or herself to a deposition or to court (Brodnik et al. 2012, 37).

128. **a** Unacceptable documentation practices include backdating progress notes or other documentation in the patient's record and changing the documentation to reflect the known outcomes of care (versus what was done at the time of the actual care). It is the HIM professional's responsibility to work with others to ensure that patient documentation is accurate, timely, and created by authorized parties. The professional Code of Ethics requires the HIM professional to assure accurate and timely documentation (Johns 2011, 778).

129. **b** Acknowledgment forms are used to document the fact that information about the patient's rights while under care was provided to the patient. Referred to as the patient's bill of rights, Medicare Conditions of Participation require hospitals to provide patients this information. The information must include the right to refuse treatment (Johns 2011, 90).

130. **d** Errors in paper-based records should be corrected according to the following process: Draw a single line in ink through the incorrect entry. Then print the word *error* at the top of the entry along with a legal signature or initials and the date, time, and reason for change and the title and discipline of the individual making the correction. The correct information is then added to the entry. Errors must never be obliterated. The original entry should remain legible, and the corrections should be entered in chronological order. Any late entries should be labeled as such (Johns 2011, 107).

131. **c**   Privacy, confidentiality, and security are related, but distinct, concepts. In the context of healthcare, privacy can be defined as the right of individuals to control access to their personal health information. Confidentiality refers to the expectation that the personal information shared by an individual with a healthcare provider during the course of care will be used only for its intended purpose. Security is the protection of the privacy of individuals and the confidentiality of health records (Johns 2011, 49).

132. **c**   Justice would require the HIM professional to apply the rules fairly and consistently for all and not to make special exceptions based on personal or organizational perspectives (for example, releasing information more quickly to a favorite physician's office) (Johns 2011, 753).

133. **a**   It is generally agreed that social security numbers (SSNs) should not be used as patient identifiers. The Social Security Administration is adamant in its opposition to using the SSN for purposes other than those identified by law. AHIMA is in agreement on this issue due to privacy, confidentiality, and security issues related to the use of the SSN (Johns 2011, 387).

134. **c**   The HIPAA Privacy Rule permits healthcare providers to access protected health information for treatment purposes. However, there is also a requirement that the covered entity provide reasonable safeguards to protect the information. These requirements are not easy to meet when the access is from an unsecured location. In addition, if the physician has access and can print or copy the information, it further increases the possibility of a violation of the regulations. To eliminate some of the risks, physicians can gain access through a dedicated portal on a secure gateway or have virtual private network (VPN) access. The covered entity may also require a physician to sign an agreement that he or she will provide reasonable safeguards to protect the information (Thomason and Dennis 2008, 28).

135. **a**   Present on admission (POA) is defined as a condition present at the time the order for inpatient admission occurs—conditions that develop during an outpatient encounter, including the emergency department, observation or outpatient surgery, are considered as present on admission. A POA indicator is assigned to principal and secondary diagnoses and the external cause of injury codes based on physician documentation (Johns 2011, 325).

136. **d**   Discounting applies to multiple surgical procedures furnished during the same operative session. For discounted procedures, the full APC rate is paid for the surgical procedure with the highest rate and other surgical procedures performed at the same time are reimbursed at 50% of the APC rate (Johns 2011, 330).

137. **d**   SNF reimbursement rates are paid according to Resource Utilization Groups, Version III (RUG-III) (a resident classification system) based on the MDS resident assessments (Johns 2011, 328).

138. **c**   Because CDI involves the medical and clinical staffs, it is more likely that the CDI project will be more successful if these staff are included in developing the process for documentation improvement. Because all hospital staff do not document in the health record, a memorandum from the CEO to all staff would not be efficient or necessarily effective. The chairperson of the CDI project does not have line authority for employee evaluation. The Joint Commission performs oversight activities but would not be involved in direct operational tasks such as this (Schraffenberger and Kuehn 2011, 360).

139. **b** An appeal is a request for reconsideration of denial of coverage for healthcare services or rejection of a claim. Second and third opinions are cost-containment measures to prevent unnecessary test, treatments, medical devices, or surgical procedures. These second and third opinions are particularly sought when test, treatment, medical device, or surgical procedure is high risk or high cost; diagnostic evidence is contradictory or equivocal; or experts' opinions are mixed about efficacy (Casto and Layman 2011, 71, 100).

140. **b** Fraud in healthcare is defined independently by a number of legal authorities, but all definitions share common elements: a false representation of fact, a failure to disclose a fact that is material (relevant) to a healthcare transaction, damage to another party that reasonably relies on the misrepresentation or failure to disclose. This situation would fall under category 2 (Brodnik et al. 2012, 430–431).

141. **b** The major components of the revenue cycle are preclaims submission activities performed by admitting and case management; claim processing activities, which is performed by multiple areas to include patient financial services and HIM coding for charge capture, Chargemaster maintenance, coding, auditing, and claims submission; accounts receivable, and claims reconciliation and collections activities performed by patient financial services (Casto and Layman 2011, 249–253).

142. **b** The charge description master (CDM) relives the coding unit of repetitive coding that does not require documentation analysis. Hard coding is the process of assigning a CPT/HCPCS code to a service so that the code will be automatically posted to the patient's account via order entry (Schraffenberger and Kuehn 2011, 228).

143. **a** Preclaims submission activities comprise tasks and functions from the admitting and case management areas. Specifically, this portion of the revenue cycle is responsible for collecting the patient's and responsible parties' information completely and accurately for determining the appropriate financial class, educating the patient as to his or her ultimate financial responsibility for services rendered, collecting waivers when appropriate, and verifying data prior to procedures/services being performed and submitted for payment (Casto and Layman 2011, 249).

144. **c** Revenue cycle began as facilities needed to structure services to meet the changing and challenging demands for reimbursement from third-party payers, compliance, patient and physician satisfaction, and demands for greater efficiencies to enhance revenue. The restructuring consisted of a realignment of departments as well as a new concept for how those departments interrelate (Schraffenberger and Kuehn 2011, 456).

145. **d** A/R refers to the charges for patient services for which the healthcare facility is awaiting payment. In other words, the third-party payers and/or patients have received the claim, but the healthcare facility has not yet been paid. Patient accounts staff members speak of A/R but rarely use the words "accounts receivable," and it is important that HIM directors and coding managers speak the same language (Schraffenberger and Kuehn 2011, 458).

146. **a** The phrase *aging of accounts* refers to the aging of the A/R after the claim has been dropped for billing. The aging "buckets," as they are often called, are usually in 30-day increments and broaden as the account gets older: 0–30, 31–60, 61–90, 91–180, 181–360, 360+. The best practice is no more than 15% to 20% of final billed A/R greater than 90 days (Schraffenberger and Kuehn 2011, 459).

147. **d** Medicare Part B medical insurance helps cover physician services, outpatient care, and home healthcare (Johns 2011, 293).

148. **d** If any changes to documentation affect the MS-DRG, the case should be rebilled. At minimum, for any MS-DRG change that indicates the hospital was reimbursed more than it should have been, the encounter should be rebilled with an explanation for the rebilling. Ultimately, the coding supervisor should determine whether the frequency of errors identified demonstrates a trend (Schraffenberger and Kuehn 2011, 319).

149. **c** Typical performance statistics maintained by the accounts receivable department include days in accounts receivable and aging of accounts. Facilities typically set performance goals for this standard. Understanding the workflow within a department is crucial for the supervisor in managing the departmental resources. To understand and control the workflow, the supervisor can perform a workflow analysis and then design the process to be more effective and efficient (Casto and Layman 2011, 253; Johns 2011, 1065).

150. **b** The accounts not selected for billing report is a daily report used to track the many reasons that accounts may not be ready for billing. This report is also called the discharged not final billed (DNFB) report. Accounts that have not met all facility-specified criteria for billing are held and reported on this daily tracking list (Schraffenberger and Kuehn 2011, 436).

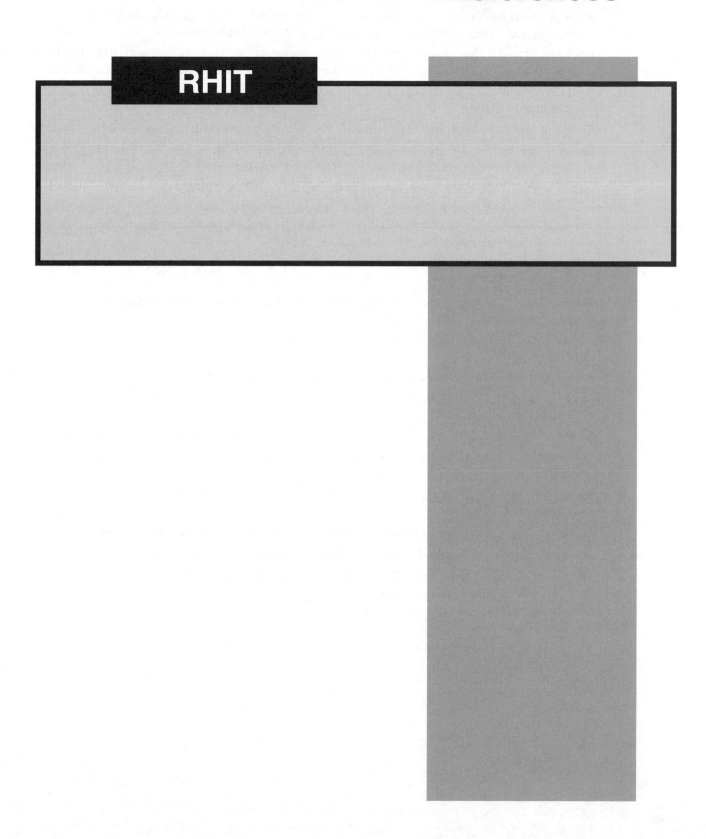

References

RHIT

References

AHIMA E-HIM Taskforce Report. 2005. Updated 2010 (Nov. 15). Practice Brief: Managing the transition from paper to EHRs. Chicago: AHIMA.

AHIMA e-HIM Work Group on Defining the Legal EHR. 2005 Practice brief: Guidelines for defining the legal health record for disclosure purposes. *Journal of AHIMA* 76(8): 64A–G.

Blackford, G. and R. Whitehouse. 2007. Getting quality clinical and coded data: How UMHS's CDIP Improved clinical coded data and clinical staff relationships. *Journal of AHIMA* 78(9): 100–102.

Brodnik, M. et al. 2012. *Fundamentals of Law for Health Informatics and Information Management*, 2nd ed., Chicago: AHIMA.

Casto A.B. and E. Layman. 2011. *Principles of Healthcare Reimbursement*. Chicago: AHIMA.

Center for Medicare and Medicaid Services (CMS). 2010 (May 21). Manual System. Pub. 100-07 State Operations Provider Certification. Transmittal 59, Section A-105. cms.gov.

Gelzer, R. et al. 2008. Copy Functionality Toolkit. Chicago: AHIMA. ahima.org.

Electronic Code of Federal Regulations, Title 42, Part 482.24 (c)(1). Amended 2012 (May 16). http://ecfr.gpoaccess.gov/cgi/t/text/text-idx?c=ecfr&sid=dc4459313be934fd78f6e61723f1d3f9&rgn=div8&view=text&node=42:5.0.1.1.1.3.4.4&idno=42.

Johns, M.L. (ed). 2011. *Health Information Management Technology: An Applied Approach,* 3rd ed. Chicago: AHIMA.

Miller, P.J. and F.L. Waterstraat. 2004. Apples to apples: using autobenchmarking to measure productivity. *Journal of AHIMA* 75(1).

Odom-Wesley, B., D. Brown, and C.L. Meyers (eds). 2009. *Documentation for Medical Records.* Chicago: AHIMA.

Russo, R. 2010. *Clinical Documentation Improvement: Achieving Excellence.* AHIMA. Chicago.

Sayles, N.B. and K.C. Trawick. 2010. *Introduction to Computer Systems for Health Information Technology.* Chicago: AHIMA.

Schraffenberger, L.A. 2011. *Basic ICD-10-CM and ICD-9-CM Coding,* 2011 ed. Chicago: AHIMA.

Schraffenberger, L.A. and L. Kuehn. 2011. *Effective Management of Coding Services.* Chicago: AHIMA.

Shaw, P. and Elliott, C. 2012. *Quality and Performance Improvement in Healthcare.* 5th ed. Chicago: AHIMA.

Smith, G.I. 2012. *Basic Current Procedural Terminology and HCPCS Coding.* Chicago: AHIMA.

Stedman's Medical Dictionary, 27th ed. 2000. Baltimore: Lippincott, Williams, and Wilkins.

Thomason, M. and J. Dennis (ed.). 2008. *HIPAA by Example.* Chicago: AHIMA.

Walsh T. 2011 (Jan. 15). AHIMA Practice Brief: Security risk analysis and management: An overview (updated). Web extra. Chicago: AHIMA.

Formulas

Hospital Statistical Formulas Used for the RHIT Exam

Average Daily Census

$$\frac{\text{Total service days for the unit for the period}}{\text{Total number of days in the period}}$$

Average Length of Stay

$$\frac{\text{Total length of stay (discharge days)}}{\text{Total discharges (includes deaths)}}$$

Percentage of Occupancy

$$\frac{\text{Total service days for a period}}{\text{Total bed count days in the period}} \times 100$$

Hospital Death Rate (Gross)

$$\frac{\text{Number of deaths of inpatients in period}}{\text{Number of discharges (including deaths)}} \times 100$$

Gross Autopsy Rate

$$\frac{\text{Total inpatient autopsies for a given period}}{\text{Total inpatient deaths for the period}} \times 100$$

Net Autopsy Rate

$$\frac{\text{Total inpatients for a given period}}{\text{Total inpatient deaths} - \text{unautopsied coroners' or medical examiners' cases}} \times 100$$

Hospital Autopsy Rate (Adjusted)

$$\frac{\text{Total hospital autopsies}}{\text{Number of deaths of hospital patients whose bodies are available for hospital autopsy}} \times 100$$

Fetal Death Rate

$$\frac{\text{Total number of intermediate and/or late fetal deaths for a period}}{\text{Total number of live births} + \text{intermediate and late fetal deaths for the period}} \times 100$$

Neonatal Mortality Rate (Death Rate)

$$\frac{\text{Total number of newborn deaths for a period}}{\text{Total number of newborn infant discharges (including deaths) for the period}} \times 100$$

Maternal Mortality Rate (Death Rate)

$$\frac{\text{Total number of direct maternal deaths for a period}}{\text{Total number of obstetrical discharges (including deaths) for the period}} \times 100$$

Caesarean-Section Rate

$$\frac{\text{Total number of Caesarean sections performed in a period}}{\text{Total number of deliveries in the period (including Caesarean sections)}} \times 100$$